MW00627498

Manhood's Morning

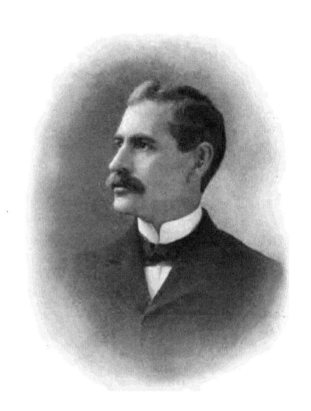

JOSEPH ALFRED CONWELL.

MANHOOD'S MORNING

A BOOK *to* YOUNG MEN *between* FOUR-
TEEN *and* TWENTY-EIGHT YEARS *of* AGE

By
JOSEPH ALFRED CONWELL

"*** *Unto you young men
because ye are strong.*"

NEW REVISED EDITION

FIFTEENTH THOUSAND

PHILADELPHIA, PA.: 1134 REAL ESTATE TRUST BLDG.
THE VIR PUBLISHING COMPANY
LONDON: 7 IMPERIAL ARCADE, LUDGATE CIRCUS, E. C.
TORONTO: WM BRIGGS, 33 RICHMOND ST., WEST

CONTENTS.

AUTHOR'S PREFACE TO REVISED
EDITION.

Few things are treasured more than our best thoughts. Time only makes them more welcome to the mind and more precious to the heart. To no one is this fact so manifest as to the one who throws his soul into a subject and after devoting days and nights to its development sends his labor forth to the world in the form of a book.

Manhood's Morning was first issued seven years ago and although lacking in typographical features it rapidly gained widespread attention. About twelve thousand copies have been published, and from every source have come hearty words of approval.

In transferring the copyright to the Vir Publishing Company the author recognizes that the book is entering upon a new career where it will secure a more extensive patronage and fill a more extended mission of usefulness.

PUBLISHER'S NOTICE.

The Vir Publishing Company herewith announce that they have secured the copyright of Manhood's Morning, by Dr. Conwell, and will in the future issue the volume in its present form. The book has been revised by the author and such changes made as new conditions require. The book in its general features, admirably blends with those already issued and will be added to our regular Series of Publications.

Dr. Joseph Alfred Conwell, the author of Manhood's Morning, was born in Delaware, forty-seven years ago, and graduated from Jefferson Medical College in 1880. In 1881 he settled in Vineland, New Jersey, where he has taken a prominent part in the church, Young Men's Christian Association and other work of public interest. Dr. Conwell is at present the Mayor of the city of Vineland, he leading the reform forces on a non-partisan ticket. Manhood's Morning is a model book

for young men and, as such, is acknowledged
to be one of the best so far issued. The volume is not a medical work. It can be read by
young women as well as by young men, and
can occupy a place on the centre-table. It
covers a wide range of subjects and is comprehensive in its scope. As a gift book to a
young man between the age of fourteen and
twenty-eight years it has no rival.

PREFACE.

Modern civilization has been richly blessed in many ways, but its chief glory has always been the strength, patriotism and character of its young manhood.

No class of individuals occupy such vantage-ground in a nation as its young men. They must, of necessity, be an essential factor in all that counts for greatness and progress.

It might be claimed that, to a certain extent, the book herein presented champions the cause of young men. No apology is deemed necessary for this feature inasmuch as the author is himself no longer young. I believe that young men are men in the highest, fullest and best sense, and that they should be so considered. No personal or selfish interests have entered into the thoughts incorporated.

There are two mistakes easily, and too often, made in writing for the young. One is to deal only with great men—famous statesmen, generals, orators, heroes, scholars and financiers—and the gigantic and wonderful in history. The other is to scribble insipid yarns and twaddle. Both are apt to do harm. Those who read either are apt to miss their

xi

place in life—one by aiming beyond it, and the other by failing to aim at all. God has a place in the world for every man—for the high and the low; for the prominent and the obscure. To fill that particular place, no matter whether it be the chief executive chair or a cobbler's bench, is the highest achievement. To aid and encourage men to seek their divinely intended sphere in life, and cheer and inspire them to do their best therein is the highest possible mission of a book.

It is not anticipated that this volume will escape criticism. Many, no doubt, will feel that too much is claimed for young men, that their sphere has been enlarged to an unwarranted scope. No innovations have been striven after. The book has been written under a firm conviction of its truth though, of course, not without a strong sense of its fallibility.

A portion of what the volume contains has formed the basis of a number of addresses delivered upon various occasions, chiefly to audiences of young men. These addresses were appreciated far beyond expectations and the numerous and pressing requests, from sources claiming my highest respect, that they be published have greatly encouraged me in sending forth the book.

The book has been written in a somewhat

fragmentary manner, here a little and there a little, and under a great variety of circumstances. Consequently, to the critical reader, it will appear somewhat disconnected and desultory. A large number of books, more or less related to the subjects in hand, have been read and studied and to their authors, too numerous to name, I cheerfully acknowledge my indebtedness. Extensive quoting has, however, been avoided and, as a rule, limited to the preludes to each chapter and an occasional verse, couplet or short extract emphasizing the thought to be conveyed. The volume is essentially a new book. It is the result of an extended and close study among young men. The world as it is, and not the thoughts written in books, has been my school. The chief aim has been to help young men to think in the right direction and inspire them with courage to walk and act accordingly. If there is a lack of charity at any point my pen has proven unfaithful to my desire.

It is a grave responsibility to send forth a book to be read and discussed by young men. The issues of life often originate over the printed page. Thousands owe their success and perhaps a greater number owe their ruin to books. Franklin said of a small volume, read when a youth: "If I have been a useful citizen the public owes the advantages of it to that little book."

One of the chapters of this volume was loaned to a family and read by one whose fortunes are yet to be made. He read it intently and when he had finished he stood up and with a countenance seriously set, and with a determined emphasis exclaimed: "I will be somebody; I am determined to be of some account in the world." May it so influence and inspire all who read its pages.

Every morning in the year, within our nation, more than fifteen hundred boys get out of bed and romp, play, sing, serve at home, study at school and make hilarious and glad city, hamlet and farm. When the shades of night settle deep over hill and valley, weary, innocent and hopeful of the morrow, they retire. They sleep and dream, view fair and enchanting visions and live in floating castles. At dawn they awake from their slumbers, arise, and, in the light of a new day, go forth, not boys or children any longer, but MEN— divinely endowed men—to begin anew the things of life—to put away childish things— to begin at the foot of the hill and aspire to its summit, to learn lessons of patience, industry, self-denial and endurance.

They go out from home into the world to meet and mingle with fifteen hundred other men one day older than themselves, and with others still older, thus forming a mighty legion —thirteen million in number—all of them young, yet men; all of them men, yet young. Together they plod and labor and press upward and on; some in high and some in humble paths; they build homes, they woo and wed and establish firesides; they sow and reap, endow the race with power and clothe the earth in beauty. Some wax strong and grow in fame; some struggle in weakness and want; some rejoice in success and health; some weep in sorrow and misfortune, and not a few fall by the wayside.

But the period of young manhood is transient. Time brings age and age claims all. With hands hardened by toil, with fortunes fixed by fate and with ranks broken by death, *manhood's morning* vanishes forever.

Thus do young men come forth and act their part, and borne by the flight of time pass on into age, where, one by one, as the years roll by, like weary and footsore travellers, they enter the final rest. As in the sleep of another childhood let it be hoped, they will rest and slumber, and at the dawn of another day, and at the music of another clime, they will awake and, redeemed and glorified arise, and go forth rejoicing, clothed in youthful beauty, like unto heaven, and as lasting as the sunshine of the eternal morning.   J. A. C.

CHAPTER I

Thirteen Million Strong

Let no man despise thy youth.

Paul.

"Not in life's ebbing twilight,
  Nor during its noontide glow;
The best of life is *manhood's morning*,
  They reap rich harvests who wisely sow."

"Among the works of man, which human life is
rightly employed in perfecting and beautifying, the
first in importance surely is man himself."

What a piece of work is man! How noble in reason! how infinite in faculty, in form, in moving how
express and admirable! in action how like an angel!
in apprehension how like a God! the beauty of the
world! the paragon of animals.

Shakespeare.

Manhood in its fresh embodiment—healthful,
strong, and majestic—and womanhood in its rosy
morning—fragrant with sweet thoughts and hopes
and radiant in its dewy beauty—attract the love and
admiration of all.

J. G. Holland.

Yield your young heart up cheerfully to the battle
of life. Calculate upon difficulty; but calculate also
upon success; only be sure you do it wisely.

Daniel Wise.

CHAPTER I.

THE Science of Man is the most difficult branch of knowledge to learn, yet of all the subjects we are called upon to investigate and study, it is the most interesting and important. The subject is so complex and comprehensive that he who undertakes to master it is apt to become bewildered by what he sees existing beyond the extreme limits of his greatest research. Although the subject is beyond complete comprehension, the fact remains that "The proper study of mankind is man."

There never was a time perhaps, in the whole history of the human race, when the lives of men were singled out individually and made subjects for study as now. Let a man acquire great wealth, become eminent in any profession or calling, or achieve greatness or fame among his fellow men, and he at once becomes a closely studied object lesson for the rest of the world. The methods of such a man become mottoes and his utterances become

19

maxims of accepted wisdom to direct and inspire others in climbing the difficult but royal road to fame and fortune. Indeed, the secret of success is the modern oracle, and he who by wisdom, wit, or genius, unfolds it in his life, secures for his name the homage and admiration of the generations of earth.

THE SUBJECT OF THIS BOOK IS MAN. The treatment of so broad a topic however, must of necessity be only partial and cannot be considered in its fullest sense. In the more modern and improved methods of study, when a subject is to be considered, it is divided and subdivided into various parts and appropriately classified in order to gain specific and definite knowledge, and fix the knowledge thus gained in the mind. In this manner the astronomer divides the stars into various systems and constellations, and classifies them according to their behavior in the heavens; the botanist divides plants into various orders or groups and classifies them still further according to special characteristics, in order to make their study both tangible and interesting.

So in the study of MAN, it is essential to divide the subject into various classifications in order to bring clearly to mind special knowledge, and to learn special lessons therefrom. As occasion requires, we select for study the different kinds and types of men; the noble and the base, the learned and the ignorant, the patriotic and the anarchal, the rich and the poor, the native born and the foreign, the thrifty and the shiftless, the industrious and the indolent, the upright and the vicious, and from any of these classes we can learn lessons both interesting and profitable.

In this book, devoted to the study of the subject of MAN, but one distinction will be named, —that of *age*,—and the subject briefly and specifically stated is

THE YOUNG MEN OF OUR NATION.

During the past few years a very great deal has been said and written about young men, and we have been taught to look upon them as comprising a distinct and separate class of individuals. Indeed it is perfectly proper and natural that they be singled out as a distinct group, because in a pre-eminent degree, they possess characteristics not applicable to any other class of individuals.

They compose a distinct and separate portion of our national greatness. The young men of America form a more exclusive and representative class than any other equal number of individuals that could possibly be selected.

That there is a period of life known as the

Manhood's Morning.

age of *"Young Manhood"* none will deny. It is a period characterized by special traits of mind and character, and fraught with special endowments, opportunities, difficulties, temptations and duties.

The questions arise—and they are important ones in this connection—"What is a Young Man?" "When does a boy become a Young Man?" and "When does a Young Man cease to be a Young Man?" "When does *'Young Manhood'* begin and when does it end?" "When is a man a man, and when is that man a young man?" "What are the peculiar features and characteristics of this age, and what are the special endowments and duties belonging to this period of life?"

When the above questions are settled, the subject of young men deepens in interest and broadens in significance. Their sphere among men and the relation they hold towards business and social affairs, towards education, religion and politics and the enterprise and activities of life in general, become subjects for discussion and settlement.

As a rule, a *boy* begins to be transformed into a *Young Man* at about the age of *fourteen* years. Occasionally the transformation begins earlier, but much more often somewhat later. Physiologists and medical writers place it between the twelfth and the eighteenth year, but

Thirteen Million Strong.

in the vast majority of cases it begins, and for all practical purposes it may be considered as beginning, at the *fourteenth* birthday.

At this period many well-marked changes take place, involving not only the physical but the intellectual and moral natures. These changes are the result of a natural development or growth, and they are so gradual that the evolution takes place in many instances quite unperceived. The voice changes from the thin piping tone to the full rich voice of manhood, the body grows more erect, the shoulders broaden and grow more nearly square; the chest expands, the muscles increase in size, firmness and strength; the hair on the head becomes coarser, and the fine downy hairs which cover the body begin to grow longer and take on more color; the hair on the face begins to show itself, first as a primitive mustache, usually of much more interest to the owner than to others, and finally a beard appears upon the face; the skin becomes coarser in texture, and thicker; the taste regarding dress and personal appearance becomes more pronounced, and thus gradually, but inevitably, the boy crosses the threshold of manhood. He is no longer a boy. He now enjoys a mental enthusiasm and moral courage inexperienced before. He becomes gallant and chivalrous. A new affinity draws him to the opposite sex. It becomes natural and pleasurable to him to associate with and protect ladies; he becomes energetic, and averse to restraint, he begins to think for himself, and to feel that he is surrounded by a new environment, actuated by new impulses and subject to new laws. He becomes restless, is desirous of choosing an avocation, is inclined to render an equivalent for what he receives and seeks independence in thought, will-power and action, There comes to life few moments more joyful and triumphant than that in which the heart swells and youth exclaims,

> "Time on my brow.hath set its seal;
> I start to find myself a man."

He is a new creature, and it is of the greatest importance to him to know and realize it. His parents may continue to call him a child, the people may call him a boy as formerly, the law may call him a minor or an infant, but God, who made him, through the magic and unerring voice of nature, has proclaimed him a *man*.

At this period parents realize that a change has taken place in their boy, and that he has entered into a new life. They begin to loosen restraint and to expect on the part of their offspring a self-assertion and desire to be and to do something. Paternal love is rewarded with new joys or confronted with a deeper and more anxious care. It is just as natural and as much a sacred duty for parents to welcome and recognize the advent of the man-life in their sons as it was to anticipate and prepare for their coming at birth.

The other extreme—the ending of the period of young manhood—is not so well marked, but it is none the less real. There are various characteristics peculiar to the period of young manhood only, which now disappear. These changes are not so closely looked for, nor are they so apparent as those which accompany the ushering in of manhood. They are consequently much less discussed. They are not hailed with the same amount of expectancy, because the eyes have ceased to look so hopefully into the future. The milestone in life's pathway which carries into the past the period of young manhood, is unwelcomed, unexpected, and as a rule unnoticed. It is marked by a partial cessation of certain pleasant hopeful ideas regarding life, in the place of which supervenes a modified conservative spirit, accompanied by an inclination to settle down and enjoy the comforts of home; poetry is turned into prose, romance is transformed into reality, fancy into fact and experiment into experience; man begins to see his shadow, the joy and the sorrow, the sweet and the bitter of life

25

have become accepted and inevitable verities, and whether man is conscious of it or not his fortunes become fixed by fate.

At this age most men can truthfully say

> "That year by year, and ray by ray
> Romance's sunlight dies away,
> And long before the hair is gray
> The heart is disenchanted."

The question arises :—When does this transformation from the period of young manhood into that which follows take place? When may it be said that a man is no longer a "Young Man?" As a rule the change takes place between the ages of twenty-five and thirty years, and it comes to every one. For all practical purposes the time may be placed at *twenty-eight years of age.* Indeed in most instances it takes place not far from this time. The changes wrought at this period of life may not affect the happiness nor the general character of the individual at all. He may live on just as light-hearted and joyful as before; his life may be filled with sunshine, and fortune may attend his every footstep, but at an unbidden hour in life, and, as a rule, not far from the age of *twenty-eight,* every man, no matter what his condition or experience may be, leaves behind him certain definite characteristics, opportunities and duties and they are gone forever. The transition is real and such an individual is no longer a genuine young man.

A definite period—a distinctive epoch of life—is embraced between these years. *The Young Men of America,* therefore may be considered to be composed of all male individuals between the ages of *fourteen* and *twenty-eight* years.

These fourteen years embrace just two links, of seven years each, in the chain of life—one link before reaching the prevailing legal age of twenty-one, and one link after the legal majority has been attained.

According to the Census of 1900, the total population of the United States was 76,303,-387, and of this number 39,059,242 were males. Almost exactly one-third of this number or 13,019,747 were young men between the ages of fourteen and twenty-eight. There are therefore at the present time in the United States 13,000,000 male children and boys under fourteen,

13,000,000 YOUNG MEN

between fourteen and twenty-eight and 13,-000,000 men beyond the period of young manhood.

This vast army of young men, taken as a whole, constitutes a distinct class of individuals, in many respects resembling each other, and in various ways interested in each other to a remarkable degree. Their natural sympathies are more uniform and mutual, and their business interests and social relations are more closely allied than those of any other similar number of individuals that now live or perhaps ever did live. While they are scattered throughout the length and breadth of three and one-half million square miles of territory, their intercourse with each other is more free, their interests and aims are more of a unit, and they are more universally in touch, through a common sympathy, than is the case with the inhabitants of the most closely populated city. They are more easily influenced by each other, and each in turn is more directly responsible for the acts and welfare of his fellows, than can be said of any other class of individuals. During this period of life, friendship and good-will are purest and most sincere, personal magnetism is at its height and the social and fraternal ties are now at their strongest.

Says the eminent Lord Brougham: "At this enviable age, everything has the lively interest of novelty and freshness; attention is perpetually sharpened by curiosity; and the memory is tenacious of the deep impressions it thus receives, to a degree unknown in after life."

During these years, opportunity is at its

Thirteen Million Strong.

flood, ambition, courage and hope heed naught but conquest and victory, care and anxiety are at the ebb; disappointment now is only discipline, failures simply stepping stones to greater success, and at this time every loyal hearted and truly courageous "Young American" should possess that kind of determination, valor, and zeal which shirks no duty, fears no obstacle, and knows no defeat.

The thirteen million young men of America are a potent factor, not only in promoting national advancement, but in shaping the world's history. They represent the greatest available power of concerted human force the world can produce. Their patriotic loyalty, moral worth, and manly strength render our land absolutely invulnerable to any and every external foe.

The latent force represented by these thirteen million young men is quite beyond mental comprehension. Were they to form in line, marching ten abreast and twelve feet apart, they would form one unbroken column 2800 miles long. Were they to clasp hands they would form two unbroken lines, reaching from the Atlantic to the Pacific ocean. If each one built a house, of the average size, the buildings would line both sides of eight streets reaching across our continent. They represent sufficient labor to dig the iron ore from the mines, manufacture it into wire, lay the foundations, and construct and complete the great New York and Brooklyn Bridge in three hours.

The great Chinese wall is the unrivalled wonder of the world's industry. It is 1259 miles long, 20 feet high, 25 feet thick, and contains 20,000 towers 40 feet square at the base and 37 feet high. It took hundreds of years to build it and it is the most stupendous structure erected by man. If laid down in the United States it would reach from Niagara Falls to Dallas, Texas, or from New Orleans to New York. It would wall our Atlantic seaboard from Nova Scotia to Florida; yet with the aid of modern machinery, the Young Men of America represent enough force to dig the clay from the earth, manufacture the bricks and construct the wall complete in five days. If they would begin to save and place at interest one dollar per week and continue to do so until sixty years of age, they would thus accumulate a sum surpassing the entire wealth of every kind and nature, both personal and real, public and private, of the United States at the present time.

For each one to be sick one day is equal to 31,000 being sick an entire year. They represent enough labor to go into the forests and hew the timbers, to go into the mines and dig the iron, and manufacture it into steel rails and spikes, and construct a railroad reaching from

Thirteen Million Strong.

New York City to San Francisco between the rising and the setting of the sun.

For each one to invest one hundred dollars, would capitalize thirteen thousand banks, each having a capital of one hundred thousand dollars. Two cents daily from each would send three hundred thousand young men to college. For each one to waste ten cents daily is equal to the destruction of three hundred and seventy-five thousand houses, costing twelve hundred dollars each, annually, or equal to reducing to ashes a town of five thousand inhabitants every day in the year.

That these thirteen million young men represent fully as much intellectually and morally as they do physically, is a fact too often overlooked. In every way they represent the dominating factor in our national make-up.

Perhaps no class of individuals is so little understood as young men. Yet no class exhibits qualities more natural and uniform.

Those older in years, under the guise of leadership and philanthropy, have spent much time trying to solve the problem as to what to do with our young men.

Young men have been looked upon as a care —as wards and dependents—in the realm of business activity and progressive civilization. The world is slow to learn, and when it is taught is quick to forget, that young men are

Manhood's Morning.

strong in muscle, mind and character, and that
they, more than any others, are capable of carrying on the world's work. Another mistake
made is, men in general and young men in particular are belittled by a low estimate being
made of their possibilities. Men are the highest expression of the Infinite Mind, and the
best kind of man is a young man. They may
be limited in their abilities, as most men are,
yet they are not on this account in any sense
insignificant. Each man, however humble in
position or limited in powers, is an essential
part of an important whole. There are stars in
the heavens which seem of little account, yet if
one were to fall it would disturb the entire
heavens. There are men, weak in influence, yet
they belong in their several places and for them
to forsake duty embarrasses society as a whole.

"What is really needed," says Gladstone, "is
to light up the spirit that is within a young
man" . . . . "There is in every young
man the material for good work in the world;
in every one, not only in those who are brilliant,
not only those who are quick, but in those who
are solid, and even those who are dull or seem
to be dull."

> "Arouse him then; this is thy part;
>   Show him the claim; point out the need,
> And nerve his arm and cheer his heart;
>   Then stand aside, and say: 'God-speed.'"

Thirteen Million Strong.

The greatest duties, the most difficult to perform—are small duties. The greatest achievements are not those historic deeds of greatness which are held up for admiration, but the small acts that are performed by the millions. As the stones for Solomon's Temple were hewn and chiseled by men in obscurity, and were brought together and piled into the magnificent structure without fault or blemish, so it is with the faithful toil and loyal lives of men to-day. The great army of America's common people, such as most young men are, is the force which hews and chisels the worthy deeds which, when taken together, make our history noble and our nation prosperous.

CHAPTER II

The Best Years of Life

Rejoice, O young man * * * and walk in the ways
of thine heart, and in the sight of thine eyes.

Solomon.

"Young man—go forth in thy strength.
  Strike out—God will lead the way;
Why wait for the noontide sun?
  Morning is the best of day."

It is with men as with plants; from the first fruits
they bear we learn what may be expected in the future.   *Demophilus.*

"In the lexicon of youth which fate reserves for a
bright manhood there is no such word as—fail."

Up, then, with a heroic spirit, and gird yourself for
mortal conflict with the great Apollyon who bestrides
your pathway! If he has subdued thousands, thousands have also subdued him. And you too may be
his conqueror!

Wise.

Why wilt thou defer thy good purpose from day to
day? Arise and begin in this very instant, and say,
Now is the time for doing, now is the time for striving, now is the fit time to amend myself.

Thomas a' Kempis.

"Ye whose cheeks are rosy bright,
  Whose hands are strong, whose hearts are clear,
Waste not of hope the morning light!
  Ah, fools; why stand ye idle here?"

36

CHAPTER II.

THROUGHOUT all history the period of young manhood has been regarded as the most intensely vital part of life. Man possesses many natural and important characteristics at this time, which give him a superior nature, and which place him at his best. As a rule, all the higher attributes which add vigor, force and attractiveness to manhood are now more prominent than at any other age. These years—from fourteen to twenty-eight—may be justly singled out as the most important, eventful and useful years of man's earthly career. Writers upon the subject have been inclined to place man's best years later in life. Such a theory however, will not stand the test of candid judgment and experience. With extremely rare exceptions, a man is as much of a man, and of far more individual importance, at twenty years of age than he is at forty. The fact that a man has acquired success, social standing, or become the father of a family, does not prove that he has grown in in-

37

Manhood's Morning.

dividual importance or worth. Just the opposite
is the truth. Such a man at forty is not render-
ing to society and to the community so great a
service as when he was striving to win and
merit what he has gained; he is not so much a
guardian and father to his children now as
when the powers which gave them existence
were within his vitals; his accumulated wealth
is not so much a part of his individual make-up
now as it was when it was stored up in his
muscle, will power and brain. The world can
spare such a man now a thousand times better
than it could when he stood the incarnation of
all these possibilities, at the threshold of manhood.

In a supreme manner the young men of a
nation are the trustees of posterity. The thirteen million young men of America, in a more
delicate and real sense, hold guardianship over
the vast legion of men and women, yet unborn, than do the millions of fathers around
whose knees prattle and play the children of our
great and populous land. The young men hold
posterity within their life powers, and are daily
moulding the character, measuring the success
and determining the moral and mental capacity
of their future offspring. They, like magic
artists, are shaping the forms and inspiring the
countenances, adding graceful curves to the
outline and brightness to the eyes, and mixing

The Best Years of Life.

the identical colors that shall paint the cheeks of their posterity for generations to come. The fathers of the nation may do whatsoever they may choose and it matters little, but the young men who represent the transmitting influences which shall some day be transformed into men and women of a still more important and exceptional age, cannot commit a good or evil deed, or even think a good or evil thought, without imparting an influence for good or evil as penetrating and as lasting as the forces of kinship and parenthood.

During this epoch of life, not only are the latent forces more profoundly impressionable, but the vital and active powers of mind and will are more tense and vigorous. The muscle is more agile and elastic, the intellect more alert and clear, the comprehension more unbiased and concentrated, the impulses more unselfish, the motives more exalted, the will more invincible, the ambition more determined, the forensic powers more magnetic, and the friendships and affections more sincere. Take him all in all, man wields a greater influence over his own nature, over his associates and upon the world at large at this time than at any other period of life.

> "Scion of a mighty stock!
> Hands of iron—hearts of oak—

39

Manhood's Morning.

Craft and subtle treachery,
Gallant youth! are not for thee."

According to authentic statistics these fourteen years from every standpoint, comprise almost exactly the middle third of life. It has
already been stated that of the 39,000,000 males
of our nation the 13,000,000 young men occupy
the central place. Again, at the age of twenty-
one—the centre of this period—the population
of the nation is divided almost exactly into two
equal portions, as there are about the same
number under twenty-one as there are over
this age. Twenty-one years of age—the centre
of this epoch—is also almost exactly the centre
of the average duration of life of the male
population of our nation at the present time.
Young men between the ages of fourteen and
twenty-eight therefore represent the central
portion—the middle third—of our male population. They form the *central pillar* of the
three great columns of life—the *zenith* between
the rise and decline, between childhood and age
—the *central links* in the chain—the *keystone*
in the arch—the *main stretch* in the race.

The fact that these years form the most useful and important epoch in life cannot be too
strongly emphasized. Those under fourteen
are in the embrace of childhood. They think

40

The Best Years of Life.

and comprehend only as children do, and are concerned in childish things. They have not begun to live in the broadest and most significant sense. The life of toiling activity which awaits them is so far a hidden mystery. They are dependent upon others for food, clothing and shelter, and manhood will be to each of them the evolution of a new creature. Those who have passed beyond the age of twenty-eight are no longer young men. They have undergone a transformation. They have, almost to a man, sealed their fate and either solved or ignored and placed beyond reach of solution the great problems of life. Their success has been established, or misfortune and fixed and settled conditions have become permanent obstacles to their progress and usefulness. Most men over twenty-eight are simply passive and slavish followers of previously formed plans and habits and permanently wrought circumstances. The future to them is simply a continuation of the past, adding a few more chapters to a volume plotted and outlined to the final page, and the chief portion written.

Those who have planned wisely and those who have planned foolishly, both find the wind and tide going their way, carrying the one to success and usefulness, the other to failure and despair.

As years pass by the evil days draw nigh

to most men, perhaps to all; wholesome interests and hopeful vigor wane, selfishness and conservative habits supervene, and the ideas and energies which once represented enterprise and progress, become fossilized and useless debris among the achievements of a new age.

Into the fourteen years, during which men are young and vigorous, the Infinite Mind has irrevocably crowded nearly all of the great and important events of life. God would not have forced men to work out so many of life's problems at this age without giving them extra powers and capabilities for effort and accomplishment. The laws of the land consider a young man simply an infant until he is twenty-one, but nature has written a law more inexorable —that manhood's duties begin earlier and they cannot be safely delayed. Legions of young men are ruined while idling away their time waiting for a legal title to manhood. A thousand make the mistake of postponing their opportunity to begin, where one begins too soon. A timely beginning is imperative in the accomplishment of life's work.

Unless young men early grasp their opportunity and are always prepared to utilize the natural but rapidly passing evolution of life's events, they fail in their mission and forfeit their usefulness.

Man, to a remarkable degree, is the architect

The Best Years of Life.

of his own fortune, and during the early years of manhood come the best and almost always the only chances to plan and construct some of the most difficult portions of life's work. Man does not grow into greatness from something insignificant, like the slow growth of an acorn into an overspreading oak—but he builds. He plans and constructs himself. He must lay the foundation—the most important part—first. He is given simply enough material to construct his fortune—with none to spare—and he is required to plan the whole structure and use the choicest materials at the very start. If he makes a mistake his loss is permanent. He must build first. Future operations are at best only additions to the original design.

At the very beginning young men must, in order to achieve success, choose their occupation—select their life work. The day has gone by when a trade or profession can be "picked up" and carried to its highest success; and the time is rapidly passing when it is possible to attain even a moderate success unless that calling is chosen for which the individual is specially adapted. Mistakes in selecting a vocation are becoming more serious. The curse of our industrial and professional systems is misfits—"round men in square holes, and square men in round holes." It is as great a sin to murder our talent as it is to bury it. "It is

43

an incontrovertible truth, that no man ever made an ill figure who understood his own talents, nor a good one who mistook them." It is pitiful to see a man in the pulpit who should be digging ditches, but it is a sin for a good preacher to spend his life shoveling dirt. God made every man for a purpose, yet a great majority of mankind upset the divine plan by thoughtlessly and carelessly drifting into some occupation for which they possess no talent or adaptation. To trifle as most young men do, over such an important matter, is a personal disgrace, and results in an enormous accumulation of industrial and business shipwrecks. To overlook natural adaptation in selecting a calling and to follow that for which one is not fitted is downright dishonesty and cowardice— it not only buries the talents, but turns work into toil and drudgery, and renders the life of the offender unnatural and artificial. They only are happy whose labor and talents harmonize. No one so demoralizes a trade, a profession or a business as the awkward misfit therein striving to succeed. The imperative need of the times is a more masterly service, and no reform will invite the millennium more surely than for every man to study his natural ability and talent and wisely follow their leadings. Untrained hands and unguided talents are a nuisance to the republic. Pauperism and

The Best Years of Life.

crime are the natural offspring of an idle, tradeless manhood. Jails and almshouses swarm
with lapsed talent and skill. The modern tramp
and the legion of failures along life's highway
are simply examples of the man who kept his
talent in a napkin. Tradeless men have no permanent grasp upon industry; the world does
not owe them a living and at best they are only
industrial ballast. Neither education, wealth
nor religion can atone for neglecting to master
a craft or business whereby to become useful
and self supporting. The chief reason why so
many young men fail to master some trade or
business and why so many who do make the
effort make a mistake in their choice, is because they do not begin early enough. As a
rule, unless it is begun before the age of twenty,
it is either never done at all or done at more
or less of a compromise of the highest possibilities.

Choosing an occupation is no small matter.
It requires that a young man honestly and intelligently measure his own ability and fitness
and act accordingly.

It belongs to every young man to know,
better than any one can tell him, what he would
like to do and what suits him best. No rules
can be written to guide him. The world's
greatest successes have often defied the most
plausible advice. There is an inward impell-

ing force, a calling of God perhaps, to every noble ambition which tends to lead in the right direction, and, as a rule, every young man must decide for himself regarding his occupation.

During these years young men must leave home. To leave the parental roof and go out into the world is the lot of most young men. The event with its accompanying experiences is entirely natural and should always lead to wholesome results. Garfield said: "Nine times out of ten the best thing that can happen to a young man is to be thrown overboard and compelled to swim or sink for himself." The world is a great school and there are lessons which give power to the will, strength to the character and fibre and force to the individual which can be learned nowhere else. It is the time and the place in which God tempers the metal and tests the faith of manhood. The best education that can come to us is obtained in our early struggles to earn an honest living—the greater the struggles the more valuable and enduring the lessons. There is much wisdom in the words of Saxe:—

"In the struggle for power, or scramble for pelf,
  Let this be your motto, 'Rely on yourself,'
For whether the prize be a ribbon or throne,
  The victor is he who can go it alone."

Never does a young man so completely hold within his grasp his fortunes and destiny as

The Best Years of Life.

when he first ventures alone upon the great battlefield of life. As a rule the pivotal step which
decides between success and failure is taken at
this time. By being thrown upon their own resources young men develop self-confidence,
industry and independence; they learn to as-
sert their own rights and to love what is theirs
because they earn it, they become broad-minded
and self-respectful and acquire moral courage.

The now famous painting, *"Breaking Home
Ties,"* by the lamented Thomas Hovenden,
which won the First Prize at the Chicago
World's Fair, represents an American boy leaving home to battle for himself. "More than a
thousand boys like this one go out from their
homes every day to make homes for themselves,
to create new conditions, to acquire property,
to marry well and establish other families, to
become good citizens and valued members of
new communities, to develop that estate of
American manhood which is the strength of
the strongest of nations." Art to such a man is
a noble thing. "He made his skill preach
homely lessons, interpret the elemental virtues
of humanity and minister to the upbuilding of
domestic purity and national honor."

> "On many a lip an honored name is heard,
> In many a hall his genius wins the prize;
> A nation's heart is touched to tender joy,
> At the sweet vision, 'Breaking Home Ties.' "

47

Manhood's Morning.

*During these years young men must estab-
lish a home of their own.* While it is allotted
to most young men to leave the home of their
birth, it is their duty to find another. Man is a
domestic being and his highest happiness is enshrined in the home; indeed the stability of our
nation is embodied in the home life of its people. Contentment seldom if ever permanently
forsakes the fireside, and when a young man
loses the love of domestic joy he forfeits the
noblest traits of citizenship. If every man in
America had a good home—where contentment, comfort and felicity abide—we would
need little law and none to enforce it. Millions
of young men are without homes. They drift
from place to place, from job to job, until, divorced from natural affections and settled motives in life, they become a national peril rather
than a tower of strength and protection. Rid
of their nobler qualities, they roam around like
vermin, consuming and destroying the most
precious elements of our social and national
greatness. Discouraged and robbed of their
natural estate they are driven hither and thither,
first by booms of industrial prosperity, then
by waves of discontent. The panacea for national discontent and business depression is not
more money but more homes. Nothing can
take the place of the family fireside, and to none
is it so beneficial as to young men. They can-

48

not begin too early to plan and build a place that
shall be to them a home, where all the hallowed
influences which add comfort, happiness, stability and character to life, shall meet and
abide.

*During this epoch of life young men must
get married.* It is the natural, divinely appointed time for this important event. During
these years a man is better qualified to fall in
love and marry than at any other time. Affection is never so pure, social ties never so
strong, and friendship never so sincere as now.
The greatest bliss that falls from heaven blesses
the man who brings genuine worth to meet its
worthy equal at the marriage altar. The highest conceptions of life recognize marriage as the
unfolding of a divine plan. At no time does
the guiding hand of our Heavenly Father come
nearer than when man and woman, drawn together by the wooing of natural adaptation and
tender affection, pledge their joys and sorrows,
and the twain are transformed into a hallowed
unit.

When a young man seeks a wife, he steps
upon holy ground and must press his claims
alone. Friendship, be it ever so loyal, can never
follow love. Cupid has a realm of his own;
none but the elect inhabit his kingdom and he
converses in a language which none others can
understand. There are millions of young men

Manhood's Morning.

in our land whose weal or woe will be sealed by the marriage vow.

The progress, the happiness, the health and the destiny of the world depend upon wise marriages. Solomon said: "Every wise woman buildeth her house," and the man who is wise marries her and lives in it and his life is a triumphant song of peace, joy and contentment.

A good woman with an unworthy husband is to be pitied; no less pitiable is a good man with an unworthy wife. The wife, more than the husband, is the maker or destroyer of not only the happiness but of the success of wedded life. Woman, more than man, is blessed with a fund of those endearing qualities which make life joyous and beautiful. It is a part of her mission to give to the home her felicitous influence. It is the very thing man most needs.

> "A perfect woman, nobly planned,
> To warn, to comfort, and command."

Man is astonishingly influenced by these things; far more than people imagine. Domestic happiness or the lack of it stamps his career with success or failure. If I am a judge, men are more impressionable than women, and more husbands than wives, on account of domestic infelicity become discouraged, and, stranded upon life's pathway, die broken-hearted. The man who marries a good wife does

50

not have to strive half so hard to get to heaven as the man who marries a bad wife does to keep out of perdition. It is a common expression that "When a woman marries it is the last of her," but it is often the beginning of the man, and upon nothing does natural prosperity and universal progress so surely depend as upon young men thoughtfully, and in proper season, entering into and cultivating all the endearments of the marriage relation.

He who fails to invoke Divine direction and approval and to follow the leadings of his own higher nature in the choice of a wife, deals a fatal blow to life's most sacred duty and blights forever the most fragrant flower that adorns its pathway.

*During these years the strategic opportunities and experiences—*THE CRISES*—of life come and go.* That "there is a tide in the affairs of men which taken at its flood leads on to fortune," is a truth almost universally accepted. Golden opportunities, no doubt, come to all, but they come but once and usually before the time expected. Opportunity comes, it is said, in the form of youth, with blushing cheeks and flowing locks, but if it finds its host unprepared, or if it be not warmly welcomed it turns, and exhibiting a bald head, it hurries away. It comes in leisurely through the front door and if not recognized, in its hurry to leave, jumps

out at the window. Real good chances of success never stand and plead at anybody's door.
That so many opportunities are allowed to pass
by is not because they come at the wrong time,
but because young men think that others will
come at a more convenient season.

To recognize opportunities requires the keen,
active and helpful faculties of the young, rather
than the conservative thoughtfulness and experience of the elderly.

Youthful ambition, with its hopefulness and
earnest zeal, is of infinitely more service in
embracing chances of success than accumulated
knowledge gained by experience, be it taught
by either past successes or failures.

Not only must opportunities be quickly
caught but preparations must be made for them
beforehand. Indeed one of the great secrets
of success is to be prepared always for a good
opportunity. There is only one secret greater
than this—the secret of making the opportunity
itself.

> "To catch Dame Fortune's golden smile
> Assiduous wait upon her."

The vicissitudes of these years are supremely
vital and important and make or unmake success. Courage, sagacity, faith and decision of
character are put to their severest tests. There
are certain times during this epoch when questions must be settled which affect the entire life,

The Best Years of Life.

and when a mistake brings a bitterness for which there is no remedy. There occasionally comes to almost every young man a supreme hour—a crisis—when life's highway seems to divide, and a choice must be made that shall shape the destinies not only of time but of eternity. Fortunate is the young man, who, at such critical moments, can rise to the full stature of his manhood, choose the right, trust in God, win the victory and triumphantly go forward. One thing is usually common in the experiences of the rich and the poor, the happy and the miserable, the saved and the lost, and that is, the little circumstances back in the past which proved stumbling blocks to one and stepping stones to the other. Success and failure often turn upon very small pivots. There is nothing more insignificant in appearance than a golden opportunity, and thousands of young men amount to little because they fail to grasp their best chance. They waste the lucky day, sleep the golden hour, wince at the crucial moment—the crisis passes by—and their highest possibilities are blighted and stranded forever.

During this period it is the duty of young men to become Christians. Nearly all who become useful Christians do so in early life. A man is seldom converted after twenty-eight; not one in ten between thirty and forty; not one in sixty between forty and fifty, and not one

53

in thrée hundred between fifty and sixty. More than 75 per cent. of those who are Christians were converted before the age of twenty-one. The Spirit which inclines the minds and hearts of men toward God and a religious life rapidly declines in influence after the age of manhood is reached. The old may be saved, but salvation is specially in behalf of the young. The Bible contains scarcely a direct promise to an aged and unconverted man, but it is full of promise to young men. To a remarkable degree it is a book about young men and for young men. Its kings, its prophets, its apostles and its heroes were chiefly young men. Jesus Christ was a young man. He experienced the vicissitudes and trials of life, and was tempted of the devil as young men only experience these things. He learned a trade, waxed strong in muscle and mind, won his own reputation among men; came in contact with the world, saw its iniquity and deception, its hypocrisy and treason in high places as young men see these things to-day. Through it all he lived a pure and blameless life. He had no experience with age, but finished his work while the glow of youthful vigor was upon his cheeks. His life is pre-eminently a pattern for young men. Nowhere is Christian character so attractive and powerful as when exemplified in the lives of young men. To none does it prove so great

The Best Years of Life.

a blessing, and to none does it give so potent an influence for usefulness.

Men must establish their habits, morals and character during these years. The acts, the desires and motives of one day become the habits and principles of the next. The lessons of ex-.perience are not only now being taught, but they must be met and profitably applied. Life's battles must be fought, temptations overcome, evils conquered, obstacles put aside and enemies overthrown.

Timothy Titcomb in his noted *Letters to Young People,* in the opening sentence to young men wrote as follows: "I suppose that the first great lesson a young man should learn is that he knows nothing; and that the earlier and more thoroughly this lesson is learned, the better it will be for his peace of mind and success in life . . . that intrinsically he is of little value." A wiser man said "The glory of young men is their strength," and "To the young man knowledge and discretion." The first great lesson for a young man to learn, the first fact to realize, is, *that he is of some importance;* that upon his wisdom, energy and faithfulness all else depends and that the world cannot get along without him. Prevailing opinions regarding the value of young men need revising. Parents, teachers, leaders of the people, business men, statesmen and rulers need educating upon this question. Parents, society and philanthropy try to do the impossible in training young men. Parents can train their children and heaven blesses the effort with a promise, but if they put off this duty until their children are men, the effort becomes unseasonable and futile. Young men must train themselves. Young men must be trusted and encouraged more, and advised and fostered less. Young men are strong physically, morally and intellectually if they are well bred, and they can plan and direct and work out their own fortunes better than anybody else can do it for them. Let us learn that God has a plan and a purpose in the life of every young man and that just as little outside advice and help as possible is desired.

Not only must young men decide the great questions of life but they must undergo the trying ordeals encountered during the early career of all undertakings. It requires more skill and energy to establish a business than it does to manipulate it later on, no matter how large it may become. The public puts young men on trial. Their workmanship, talents and integrity are weighed in the balance of popular inspection. Their reputation must be formed. They must now decide whether they will, as did the youth in "Excelsior," face life's difficulties and press on to victory, or drift with the tide and wind by following the crowd.

The Best Years of Life.

Each succeeding generation of young men finds the duties of life more difficult to perform than their fathers did. The world is constantly growing wiser and more tensely organized, and each new generation of workers must be wiser, more expert and sagacious. Young men must not only be more accomplished than their fathers are, but more accomplished than their fathers ever were. I write this reverently but candidly. In a progressive age, like the present, every branch of human activity rapidly improves, and the level to which men must aspire—or fail—is constantly being raised. The young man who mimics the methods of others, treads in the footsteps of his father, or "waits for the old gentleman's shoes," seldom succeeds.

The work and progress of the world grow more confusing and dazzling. A revolution is constantly going on—a revolution which throws men out of work and takes bread out of the mouths of children; that crushes the weak and destroys the thoughtless. Each succeeding generation of young men belongs to a new age, crowded with new conditions and subject to new laws and modes of action. It is said that the wisdom of Plato was so advanced that it took twenty centuries for the world to absorb it. If a Plato lived at the present day the world would travel at his heels. Our most brilliant

Manhood's Morning.

thinkers and inventors not only find the people
with them, but most of them find it difficult to
maintain priority in claiming the fruits of their
genius. It is a fatal delusion for young men to
conclude that the world owes them a living and
that somehow in some way it will come to them
without its equivalent in work which brings
into action their brightest faculties and best energies.

*During these years man is most capable of
performing heroic deeds and overcoming obstacles.* Faith and hope are strong and the
courage invincible. He neither looks backward
into the past nor into the future. He lives *now*,
and life is a living, present reality. Sickness
and death are least to be feared, duty and opportunity have but one watchword and its key-
note is *now*. The beauty and power of manly
vigor are now enthroned.

Young men wield a greater influence upon
society, politics and religion during these years
than do those older in years. Their personality
is more forensic and their sympathies more
spontaneous and enduring. Wealth, position
and authority may wield a power more profound, but it is autocratic and lifeless, and receives only slavish servitude. The leadership of
young men, on the other hand, is inspiring and
their dauntless courage and enthusiasm are an
incentive to our best energies. Their advent

The Best Years of Life.

brings new life into the channels of enterprise, and by their presence every phase of activity is filled with renewed confidence and vigor.

The world needs to be taught that the term *"young"* when applied to man is not intended to narrow and limit but to magnify and augment his significance. The prefix "young" is the insignia of beauty, strength and force. Young men are strong in body, mind and spirit. They represent, in the fullest measure, power of intellect, of will and of character. They impersonate natural and potent qualities, which experience cannot guide and which age will fail to improve. Added to their strength are enthusiasm, hope, purity and love, and when these attributes are properly developed and blended men become capable of the highest duties and noblest aspirations. Now is it possible to

"Wake the strong divinity of soul,
That conquers chance and fate."

Young men have been the chief actors—the impelling force—in the world's history. In their normal sphere they are the proteges of none, the protectors of all. To a remarkable degree it is true that young men have founded kingdoms, empires and republics, and formulated laws and systems of government. They have championed the world's reforms, fought its battles and turned its contests into victories.

59

They have willingly poured out their blood in the world's conflicts and given their lives as a sacrifice upon the altars of justice, liberty and truth. They have, through discoveries and inventions, kept the wheels of progress busy and turned the world into a thriving mart of commerce. They have penetrated the hidden domains and opened up a pathway for human habitation. They have founded the world's religions, overthrown its superstitions and false teachings and carried the lamp of civilization into the dark corners of the globe and spread broadcast the truths of Christian enlightenment.

CHAPTER III

What Some Young Men Have Done

Neglect not the gift that is in thee.—*Paul.*

"The heights by great men reached and kept
    Were not attained by sudden flight,
But they, while their companions slept,
    Were toiling upward in the night."

The crowning fortune of a man is to be born with
a bias to some pursuit, which finds him in employment and happiness.—*Emerson.*

Be what nature intended you for, and you will succeed; be anything else and you will be ten thousand
times worse than nothing.—*Sidney Smith.*

"Our ideals become a power upon us for the eleva-
tion of our life."

Don't flinch, flounder, fall nor fiddle, but grapple
like a man. * * * A man who WILLS it can go
anywhere and do what he determines to do.—*John
Todd, D. D.*

To wish is of little account; to succeed you must
earnestly desire; and this desire must shorten thy
sleep.—*Ovid.*

The longer I live, the more I am certain that the
great difference between men—between the feeble and
the powerful, the great and the insignificant—is
energy, invincible determination, a purpose once fixed,
and then, *death or victory.*
                                Sir Foxwell Buxton.

"For the grandest times are before us
    And the world is yet to see
The noblest work of this old world
    In the men that are to be—"

62

CHAPTER III. ·

GEORGE ˙ WASHINGTON, whose name will always stand first in our nation's history, sat down and wrote out one hundred and ten maxims of civility and good behavior for his own personal use when a boy of thirteen. He was busily engaged in surveying the wilds of Virginia at eighteen, and was an adjutant-general with the rank of major at nineteen. He fired the first gun in the French and Indian War of 1754, and commanded a regiment against the French before he was twenty-two.

LA FAYETTE, the French general and patriot, was not yet twenty when he was appointed a major-general by the American Congress, and when he fought the battle of Monmouth, for which he received a national vote of thanks, he was only twenty-one. When he revisited and made a tour of the United States he was only twenty-seven.

ALEXANDER THE GREAT spent his boyhood in diligently studying under the tutorage of Aristotle and other distinguished teachers. He

· 63

won his first battle at eighteen and ascended
the throne of Macedon as king at twenty. He
was at the head of forty thousand well disciplined troops, and defeated Darius at twenty-
two. One year later he almost annihilated the
Persian army numbering six hundred thousand men.

HANNIBAL, one of the greatest military com-
manders of any age, swore an eternal hostility
to Rome at nine years of age, and kept his vow
with the strictest fidelity. He had become the
commander-in-chief of the army at twenty-six,
having displayed extraordinary military genius
by winning several battles, and had completed
the subjugation of Spain while in his twenties.

NAPOLEON began the study of military tactics at ten; was a sub-lieutenant at sixteen, and
rapidly rose in military distinction. He was at
the head of the army of Italy, and had defeated
four of the armies of Austria at twenty-eight;
he was master of France and Europe while yet
in his twenties.

CHARLES V. was one of the most powerful
rulers and warriors of Europe before he was
twenty-five. He ascended the throne of Spain
at sixteen and at once became the most powerful ruler of Europe. At twenty he was
crowned Emperor of Germany.

LOUIS XIV. ascended the throne at five, declared himself of age at thirteen, and his court

was the centre of art, literature and science before he was twenty-one.

DAVID FARRAGUT, the noted American Admiral, entered the navy as a midshipman when only nine years of age, and was a lieutenant at twenty-one.

DEMOSTHENES and CICERO, the two greatest orators of ancient times, both dedicated their lives to oratory during childhood, and by indefatigable effort they both achieved a renown as immortal as human language while yet in their twenties. At twenty-five Demosthenes was the greatest orator of Greece, and Cicero at the same age was the greatest orator of Rome.

DANIEL WEBSTER, the eminent American orator and statesman, was such a sickly child that it was not thought that he would live, yet as a boy he had within him the elements of greatness. One day when he was about ten years of age, while sitting with his father on a hay-cock under an elm tree on the old New Hampshire farm, his father said to him: "Exert yourself—improve your opportunities—and when I am gone, you will not need to go through the hardships which I have undergone." The ten year old Daniel threw himself upon his father's breast, and as he sobbed aloud, he registered a vow, deep in his heart, that he would never idle away a moment that could be devoted to study. When he went to

Manhood's Morning.

school he was so shy that it was impossible for him to speak pieces, yet by perseverance he conquered his timidity. He had read six books of Virgil, and entered Dartmouth College at fifteen. He delivered an oration on the Fourth of July to the people of Hanover when he was eighteen years of age, of which Henry C. Lodge, his biographer said: "The enduring work which Mr. Webster did in the world, and his meaning and influence in American history, are all summed up in that boyish speech at Hanover which preached love of country, the grandeur of American nationality, fidelity to the constitution as the bulwark of nationality, and the necessity and the nobility of the union of the States." He had won fame as a lawyer, statesman and orator while yet in his twenties, and his father lived to reap the reward of his paternal devotion.

WILLIAM WILBERFORCE, the English philanthropist and champion of freedom, began his anti-slavery efforts before he was sixteen years of age, by writing an article for a paper of York, entitled, *In condemnation of the odious traffic of human flesh.* He was a member of Parliament before he was twenty-one.

WILLIAM E. GLADSTONE, the "Grand Old Man" of England, was a member of the House of Commons at twenty-three, and Lord of the Treasury at twenty-six, and it was during these

What Some Young Men Have Done.

early days as much as in later years that he immortalized his name as a financier, statesman and patriot.

THOMAS JEFFERSON was enjoying extraordinary success as a lawyer, and was a member of the Virginia House of Burgesses at twenty-six. He wrote the Declaration of Independence before he was old enough to act as President of the new nation it was intended to represent.

ALEXANDER HAMILTON, the eminent American statesman, when eighteen years of age, and about the time Great Britain and the Colonies began to disagree, wrote a number of articles in favor of American liberty, which were so patriotic and profoundly logical that their authorship was attributed to John Jay, who was a prominent American statesman and ripe scholar at the time. Hamilton was General Washington's aid-de-camp and his most trusted and confidential adviser at the age of twenty. He served in the Revolutionary war as colonel, became one of the most eminent lawyers in the State of New York and was a member of the Continental Congress at twenty-five; aided by James Madison, he took a chief part in drafting the *Constitution of the United States* while yet in his twenties.

JOHN TYLER, the tenth President of the United States, entered William and Mary College at twelve, and graduated at seventeen; was admitted to the bar at nineteen and immediately entered upon a large practice. He became a member of the State Legislature at twenty-one and entered Congress at twenty-six.

AUGUSTUS CAESAR, one of the mighty men of Rome, delivered an oration when only twelve years of age. He received the toga virilis at sixteen, and his efforts are among the most brilliant that history records, and all before he was of legal age.

WILLIAM PITT, the classical scholar and statesman, began to prepare himself for the British Parliament when nine years of age, and he was a member of that body at twenty-two. He was Chancellor of the Exchequer at twenty-three; Lord of the Treasury and Prime Minister at twenty-four; and at twenty-five he was practically the ruler of England and was acknowledged to be, at this time, the greatest master of the whole science of parliamentary government that ever lived.

LORD BACON, the philosopher and Chancellor of England, and one of the most profound scholars the world has ever produced, began to antagonize the philosophy of Aristotle when only fifteen years of age. During his boyhood, his genius and profound mental insight won universal attention. He was appointed Consul to the Queen at twenty-eight.

What Some Young Men Have Done.

PLATO, the celebrated Greek philosopher, spent his boyhood in writing poetry, but threw his verses in the fire and dedicated his life to the study of philosophy at twenty. He rapidly became one of the most profound thinkers the world has produced.

SIR ISAAC NEWTON began early in life to make his discoveries. When seated in his garden at Woolsthorpe, he saw the fall of the apple which resulted in the discovery of the laws of gravitation, and immortalized his name, he was only twenty-three. He had constructed, while yet in his teens, a clock that ran by water power; a sun-dial which remained for over two centuries on the corner of the house in which he lived, and a wind grist-mill which was so perfect that it would grind wheat into flour.

BENJAMIN FRANKLIN, the philosopher and statesman, began to write for publication when a boy of fourteen. He was publisher and editor of a newspaper, author of "Poor Richard's Almanac" and had founded the Philadelphia Public Library before he was twenty-six.

D'ALEMBERT, the distinguished French mathematician, published his first *Treatise on Dynamics,* which marked a new era in mechanical philosophy, at twenty-five.

GAUSS, one of the world's greatest mathematical scholars, devoted his early life to his favorite study and at twenty-one, was at work

69

Manhood's Morning.

upon the great arithmetic which was published two years later and which made him famous.

PASCAL, the eminent French philosopher, without the aid of books or a teacher, solved various geometrical problems upon the floor of his mother's kitchen with a piece of charcoal before he was eight years of age, and in this manner had become proficient in geometry at twelve. He invented a calculating machine, and established the theory of atmospheric pressure, and published a treatise upon the subject at twenty-five.

SIR HUMPHREY DAVY, the greatest chemist the world has produced, and the discoverer of many of the chemical elements, began the study of natural philosophy when a boy. He made his first experiments in chemistry at nineteen, and discovered the exhilarating effects of nitrous oxide, "Laughing Gas," at twenty-one. He was appointed Professor in the Royal Institution of London at twenty-two, and was the leading chemist of the age while yet a young man. He published his *Essays on Heat and Light* at twenty-one; and, in the language of Dr. Paris, "his youth, his natural eloquence, his chemical knowledge, his happy illustrations and well conducted experiments, excited universal attention and unbounded applause" at the age of twenty-three.

MICHAEL FARADAY, the distinguished Brit-

What Some Young Men Have Done.

ish physicist, was born the son of a poor blacksmith, but devoted his life to study. Hearing
Sir Humphrey Davy deliver some lectures on
chemistry, he turned his attention toward that
science and was chemical assistant in the Royal
Institute at twenty-two, and rapidly became one
of the greatest experimental philosophers the
world has ever produced.

GALILEO, who gave to the world so many
valuable discoveries, and whose name was made
immortal by the invention of the telescope, and
who was imprisoned and lost his eyesight for
saying that the earth revolved, spent his boyhood in diligent study and research. He was
only eighteen years of age when he stood in the
cathedral of Pisa and noticed how regularly the
great hanging lamp swung to and fro, and by
comparing it with the beat of his pulse he decided the accuracy in time of its movements,
from which he became the inventor of the clock
pendulum.

GAY-LUSSAC, one of the most eminent physi-
cists of modern times, began his investigations
when a boy. He published his work on *The
Dilation of Gases and Vapors* at twenty-three,
and was chosen by the French Institute to test
the magnetic force of the atmosphere, and made
a balloon ascension of more than 23,000 feet,
at twenty-six.

LORD HENRY BROUGHAM, the British states-

man, orator and scientist, was a brilliant scholar while yet in his teens. He published his
Refraction and Reflection of Light at the age
of seventeen, and was one of the founders of the
Edinburgh Review at twenty-three.

LINNAEUS, one of the world's most noted
naturalists, manifested a profound love for the
study of botany when a boy. At twenty he
was preparing a work on the *Plants of the
Bible* and prosecuting the study of medicine.
He was a successful teacher of botany and had
published his botanical work, *Hortus Uplandi-
cus*, at twenty-four.

PROFESSOR AGASSIZ, the eminent and greatly
beloved naturalist and scientist, began his favorite studies at eleven years of age, and pur-
sued them diligently during the remainder of
his life. He was recognized as one of the most
profound scholars of the age while yet in his
twenties.

HUMBOLDT, to whom physical science is more
indebted than any man of modern times, began
his studies while yet in his teens. He published
his first volume at twenty-one, and was famous while yet a young man.

JOHN J. AUDUBON, the world's greatest or-
nithologist, began the study of birds when a
youth. He was born in Louisiana but was
studying painting in Paris, at the age of fourteen as a student of the celebrated painter,
David.

What Some Young Men Have Done.

HENRY CAVENDISH, the English naturalist and chemist founded the principles of pneumatic chemistry, and discovered the element hydrogen while yet in his twenties.

SIR WILLIAM ROWAN HAMILTON, the eminent mathematician, had learned thirteen different languages at thirteen. He had thoroughly mastered all the branches of the ordinary university course and was making original investigations in mathematics, philosophy and metaphysics at fifteen. He was appointed to the chair of Astronomer Royal for Ireland at twenty-two. When he entered college as a student he presented an essay written in fourteen different languages, and during his course at college won every prize open to competition both in classics and in science. His discoveries and investigations in mathematics and the sciences made him famous while yet in his twenties.

DR. THOMAS YOUNG, the English scientist, philosopher and scholar, began his brilliant career at a very early age. He was in the Stapleton Boarding School at seven, and had acquired a remarkable knowledge of Greek, Latin and mathematics, had learned French and Latin without a teacher, and had made considerable progress in Arabic, Persic and Hebrew at fourteen. At this time a noted educator was employed to instruct him, but Young proved to

73

be more learned than his teacher. He had not only learned to speak and write various Oriental and European languages with great ease and fluency, but had gained a profound knowledge of botany, zoology, chemistry, music, natural philosophy and higher mathematics, and was studying medicine while yet in his teens. It is said of him by Rev. W. H. Milburn, "He may be styled, without exaggeration, the most learned, profound, and variously accomplished scholar and man of science that has appeared in our age,—perhaps in any age." Helmholtz, the eminent scholar and philosopher, said, "I consider him the greatest man of science that has appeared in the history of this planet." * * * "The greatest discovery I ever made was the genius and talent of Thomas Young." Professor Tyndall regarded him as immeasurably above any man that had lived since Sir Isaac Newton. While a student on his way to Gottingen University he visited Erasmus Darwin, who said of him, "He unites the scholar with the philosopher, and the cultivation of modern arts with the simplicity of ancient manners." Although a statute prohibited the granting of diplomas, except after six years' study, when he entered the College of Physicians, he was introduced by the head of the institution, Dr. Farmer, as capable of occupying any professorship in the college—"a pupil capable of reading lectures to his preceptors." At the same time he had profound knowledge of a great variety of languages and no less than fifteen of the most progressive sciences of the age. His knowledge of music was such that only one or two instruments existed that he could not play. He was an accomplished artist and one of the greatest art critics of his day. While yet in his twenties he was professor of natural philosophy at the Royal Institution, had published his *Syllabus on Natural and Experimental Philosophy, Outlines of Light and Color, Outlines and Experiments Respecting Sound and Light, Experiments and Calculations Relative to Science of Physical Optics,* and was delivering his remarkable lectures on mechanics, hydrostatics, hydrodynamics, acoustics and optics, astronomy, the theory of the tides, properties of matter, cohesion, electricity, magnetism, the theory of heat and climatology, forming the most comprehensive system of natural philosophy ever published in England. Dr. Young was one of the deepest thinkers and most profound scholars the world has produced. His motto was: "What others have done, I can do."

McCormick had conceived in his own mind, and constructed with his own hands, a harvesting reaper before he was twenty-two.

Elias Howe gave to the world one of its

greatest civilizing agents, the sewing machine, when he was a young man of twenty-six.

ELI WHITNEY, a Yankee school teacher, while yet in his twenties, invented the cotton-gin which doubled the wealth of the Southern States. Lord Macaulay said of Eli Whitney: "What Peter the Great did to make Russia dominant, Eli Whitney's invention of the cotton-gin has more than equalled in its relation to the power and progress of the United States."

DR. THOMAS MORTON gave to the world, at the age of twenty-six, what has proven to be one of the greatest blessings bestowed upon mankind—the discovery of the use of ether as an anæsthetic to relieve pain during surgical operations.

THOMAS A. EDISON, the greatest living genius, at the age of twenty-three, "penniless, friendless and hungry" made his first discovery in telegraphy, and in a very short time he was employing hundreds of men to construct the conceptions of his wonderful mind. The Commissioner of Patents styled him "the young man who keeps the path to the Patent Office hot with his footsteps." He was acknowledged to be a modern intellectual wonder while yet a young man.

ROBERT FULTON, the inventor of steam navigation, constructed paddle-wheels to a fishing boat that turned with a crank, at fourteen. He was apprenticed to a jeweler when a boy, but by selling pictures which he painted at odd hours he bought a farm for his mother and was in Europe studying art and earning his own way at twenty-one.

JOHN ERICSSON, the distinguished engineer and inventor, had made numerous drawings and mechanical contrivances, showing remarkable inventive genius, before he was eleven years of age. Among other things he had constructed a miniature saw-mill with his own hands and by his own plans. At eleven years of age he was appointed leveler at the grand Swedish canal then being constructed, and at fourteen he was appointed to set out a section, employing six hundred men. He invented a copper plate engraving machine at twenty, and a condensing flame engine at twenty-two. These were followed by an instrument for sea sounding, a hydrostatic weighing machine, a number of improvements in tubular boilers, an artificial draft by centrifugal fan blowers, and a self-acting gun lock. His celebrated steam-carriage, which made thirty miles an hour and which contained four important features of the modern locomotive, was built by him when he was only twenty-six.

GEORGE STEVENSON, the inventor of the locomotive, began to apply himself diligently to the study of steam engines when a boy of fifteen, and the history of his early years is a rare record of the complete victory of patience and perseverance over poverty and embarrassments.

SAMUEL COLT invented the revolver which bears his name, at twenty-one.

JAMES WATT, the Scotch mechanic, scientist and engineer, who, more than any one else deserves the honor of inventing the steam engine, had become such an expert, that at twenty-one he was appointed mathematical instrument maker to the University of Glasgow. He had begun his investigations into the power and capabilities of steam as a motive force before he was twenty-three, and at twenty-seven, he was working in earnest upon his wonderful improvements of the steam engine. Watt was regarded by the poet Wordsworth as "perhaps the most extraordinary man Scotland ever produced."

SAMUEL COMPTON, of Lancashire, England, to whom woman owes an everlasting debt of gratitude for inventing the spinning machine, began to sit up nights at the age of twenty-one to construct the machine that was already in his mind, and for years he labored upon it while others slept, and gave it to the world when he was twenty-six.

EDWARD GIBBON, the English historian, and in some respects, the most brilliant recorder of

What Some Young Men Have Done.

events the world has produced, began his studies, which resulted in his unrivaled historical works, at the age of seventeen, and his writings, exhibiting all the characteristics of a mature and profound scholar, began to be published when he was only twenty-four.

MULLER, the eminent Swiss historian, was Professor of Greek at twenty, and wrote his first work, *Bellum Cimbricum,* at this time. He delivered his celebrated lectures at twenty-six on *Universal History,* afterward published in twenty-four volumes.

GEORGE BANCROFT, the eminent American statesman and historian, entered Harvard College at thirteen, was made Doctor of Philosophy at the University of Gottingen at twenty, and three years later began to collect material for his wonderful masterpiece—*Bancroft's History of the United States.*

JOSEPHUS, the famous Jewish historian, was recognized as an authority upon the subject of Jewish law at the age of fourteen. He became a Pharisee at nineteen, and at twenty-six went to Rome and succeeded in obtaining the release of a number of prisoners who had been incarcerated by Felix, the same that had "trembled" before the eloquence of the Apostle Paul.

NEANDER, the celebrated ecclesiastical historian of Germany, was a profound student of theology at ten years of age, and was Professor

79

Manhood's Morning.

Extraordinary in the Heidelberg University at twenty-three.

EDWARD EVERETT, the American patriot, orator and scholar, entered Harvard College at the age of thirteen; graduated with the highest honors at seventeen; was Professor of the Greek Language and Literature in his Alma Mater, and one of the most eloquent and forceful speakers in the United States at the age of twenty.

WASHINGTON IRVING, the American author and humorist, was a classical scholar and had traveled through many foreign countries and been admitted to the bar at twenty-three. He published *Salmagundi* at twenty-four, and his *History of New York, by Diedrich Knickerbocker,* which proved to be one of the most popular books of the language, was published at the age of twenty-six.

VICTOR HUGO, one of the leading poets and novelists of modern times, was busy with his pen while yet in his teens. He published his *Odes and Ballads* at twenty, and he became famous while young in years. He was the prime mover in the literary revolution before he was twenty-eight.

·JOHN RUSKIN, one of the literary lights of the nineteenth century, was a graduate of Oxford, had won the Newdigate prize by writing poetry, had begun his independent studies in

What Some Young Men Have Done.

theology and architecture, was a recognized authority on the latter subject, had traveled extensively in England and on the Continent and had written his famous *Modern Painters*, at twenty-four.

ELIHU BURRETT, the "learned blacksmith," of New Britain, Connecticut, "sat down night after night, with aching limbs and barnacled hands," and, by patient application, mastered fifty different languages before he was twenty-seven.

BAYARD TAYLOR, the American traveler, poet and writer, was studying Latin, French and Spanish at fourteen; was teaching at fifteen. At sixteen he wrote in his Diary: "I, a humble pedagogue, might by unremitted and arduous intellectual and moral exertion become a light, a star, among the names of my country. May it be!" He began his public literary career at seventeen. His first book was published when he was nineteen. He was traveling through Europe on foot at twenty, published his *Views A-foot* at twenty-one, and was editor of the *New York Tribune* at twenty-four.

RUFUS CHOATE, America's greatest jurist, whose name will ever be the synonym of a "thorough patriot, an accomplished and profound scholar, and a gentleman of fascinating manners, of a most affectionate temper and of unsullied honor," had exhausted the town library of Essex, near where he lived, at the age of ten.

JOHN WESLEY, the founder of Methodism, practically began his life's work when a boy of eleven, by his systematic study at the Charterhouse School in London. At sixteen he was in Christ's Church College, Oxford, and soon became an exceptionally brilliant classical scholar. It was while at college that he and his brother, Charles Wesley, formed the *Holy Club*, the members of which, designated *Methodists*, proved to be the germ of one of the most powerful religious movements in the world's history. He was a polished writer and a skillful and thoughtful logician at twenty-three, and was Professor of Greek at twenty-four.

GEORGE FOX, the originator of the Society of Friends, known as "Quakers," conceived the ideas upon which their religion is based at the age of twenty-two, and began to organize and proselytize at twenty-six.

CONFUCIUS, the Chinese philosopher, spent his boyhood in diligent study and research, and married at nineteen. He was superintending public affairs at twenty. He began his theological teachings, which have shaped the religious belief of nearly one-third of the human race for over twenty-three centuries, when he was a young man of twenty-two.

MARTIN LUTHER, the leader of the Reformation, spent his early years in diligent study, and was a Professor of Philosophy at twenty-five. When he ascended the *Scala Santa* in Rome on his knees and heard the inward voice, "The just shall live by faith," he was only twenty-seven.

PHILIP MELANCHTHON, Martin Luther's fellow laborer in the Reformation, graduated from the University of Heidelberg at fifteen and from Tübingen at seventeen; had published a grammar and was Professor of Greek at Wittenberg at twenty-one. He published the first great Protestant work on dogmatic theology at the age of twenty-four, and so popular did it become that it passed through fifty editions during the author's lifetime.

JOHN CALVIN, the founder of Presbyterianism, was appointed to a benefice in the Cathedral of his native town at twelve years of age, and was given a pastoral care at seventeen. He became deeply absorbed in the study of law, theology and the languages while in his teens, at the same time teaching and preaching. He began to teach the doctrines which form the basis of the Presbyterian belief early in his twenties; his sermons were publicly burned at twenty-three, and he published his famous *Institutes of the Christian Religion* at twenty-seven.

GEORGE WHITEFIELD, the eminent preacher

83

and founder of "Calvinistic Methodism," was a boot-black, but began to write sermons during his boyhood and at twenty-one was one of the most powerful and popular pulpit orators the world has produced.

JEREMY TAYLOR, one of the greatest names in the English Church, was the son of a barber; entered college at thirteen and at eighteen was preaching in St. Paul's Cathedral in London to large and spellbound audiences.

DWIGHT L. MOODY, at seventeen, when sleeping in the gallery of a Boston church, was punched in the ribs by an old gentleman and told to "listen to the sermon." He was thoroughly awake and trying to preach at eighteen. He had become one of the most successful evangelists of the century while yet in his twenties.

CHARLES H. SPURGEON, the famous pulpit orator, was preaching at sixteen. He rapidly won fame as the "Boy Preacher" and he began to preach in the great London Tabernacle at twenty.

REV. F. E. CLARK was yet in his twenties when he founded the Young People's Society of Christian Endeavor, which now encircles the globe and has over forty-two thousand societies and two and one-half million members.

GEORGE WILLIAMS, the English dry goods

clerk, founded the Young Men's Christian Association at the age of twenty-three.

WILLIAM CULLEN BRYANT was translating Latin poems into English at ten years of age. He composed *The Spanish Revolution* and the *Embargo* at thirteen, and his celebrated *Thanatopsis* at eighteen.

ALFRED TENNYSON, late poet laureate of Great Britain, published his first verses at eighteen. He won the Chancellor's medal at Cambridge University at twenty, and a volume of poems of his own composing was published during the same year.

ROBERT SOUTHEY, the poet laureate of England, began to write verses when a mere boy and was famous at eighteen. He was poet, scholar, antiquary, critic and historian, and was a more prolific writer than Sir Walter Scott. He is said to have burned more verses before he was thirty than he published during his whole life.

JOHN MILTON, author of *Paradise Lost*, composed that exquisite poem, *Lines to a Fair Infant*, at seventeen, and his *Hymn on the Nativity*, the grandest religious lyric poem in any language, at twenty-one.

DANTE, the illustrious Italian poet, claimed to have received his poetic inspiration at nine years of age. In early life he became versed in philosophy, theology and Latin, and skillful in painting, music and other arts; he composed his celebrated *Vita Nuova* at twenty-five.

JOHN GREENLEAF WHITTIER worked on a farm and at shoemaking until he was eighteen, but by close application to study he became editor of *The American Manufacturer* at twenty-two, and of the *New England Review* at twenty-three, and rapidly won distinction and affection.

LONGFELLOW entered Bowdoin College at fourteen, and at this time began his poetical career. He was appointed Professor of Modern Languages and Literature at nineteen, and he was in the front rank of the great living poets at the age of twenty-six.

EDGAR ALLAN POE published his first volnme of poems at twenty.

JAMES MONTGOMERY, the Scottish poet, began to write poems when he was ten years of age and had composed three volumes when he was only twelve.

ALEXANDER PETOFI, the national poet of Hungary, at the age of twenty-one walked from his home to the city of Pesth, a distance of nearly two hundred miles, wearing shoes padded with straw, carrying the manuscript of a volume of poems in his bosom and two borrowed florins in his pocket. Within a few weeks he was surrounded by friends and fortune, and his verses were in wonderful de-

What Some Young Men Have Done.

mand. During his lifetime he composed 1775 poems, most of them being written while he was a young man.

THOMAS MOORE, the Irish poet, began to write for the magazines at fourteen and composed his first volume of poems while yet in his teens.

JOSEPH ADDISON, the poet and greatest of English essayists, distinguished himself in Latin verse at sixteen and was receiving a pension from the public treasury for his poetical productions at twenty-three.

ROBERT BURNS was a literary genius at twelve years of age, and a gifted poet at sixteen.

LORD BYRON published his first volume of poems while yet in his teens and was recognized as one of the most gifted and brilliant poets of the times and was a member of the House of Lords before he was twenty-five.

THOMAS GRAY began his *Elegy Written in a Country Church Yard,*—considered by many as the most finished poem in the English language—at the age of twenty-six.

THOMAS CAMPBELL, the eminent Scottish poet, was a distinguished classical scholar while yet in his teens and published *The Pleasures of Hope,* the best poem he ever wrote, at twenty-two.

JUNIUS BRUTUS BOOTH, the great American

actor, was upon the stage when seventeen years old, and he was one of the most famous tragedians of the times at twenty-one.

EDWIN BOOTH, who did more than any other man to raise the moral tone of modern dramatic art, went upon the stage when a mere boy and was playing *Richard III.* at sixteen.

SHERIDAN, the Irish dramatist and orator, was pronounced a dunce when a boy at school by his teacher, and gave no evidence of talent, but he awoke from his mental stupidity and produced his famous comedy, *The Rivals,* at twenty-four, and his still more famous production, *The School for Scandal,* was performed in Drury Lane Theatre when he was only twenty-six.

BEETHOVEN, the great composer, whose influence wrought a new epoch in music, created astonishment by his performance upon the violin at eight years of age. He played the music in Bach's *Wohltemperirtes Klavier* at eleven, and published a volume of songs and sonatas of his own composing in his thirteenth year. His fame was world-wide while he was yet in his teens.

MOZART, the immortal musician, played the clavi-chord at four years of age and composed a number of minuets and other pieces, still extant. His talents were remarkably brilliant at seven, and he took part at sight in a trio of

88

stringed instruments and gave concerts with great success in London and Paris. His achievements and fame increased with remarkable rapidity, so that at the age of thirteen years the enthusiasm and honor given him were without a parallel in the world's history.

HANDEL was composing a cantata in eight parts every week when he was only eight years of age and he produced his great opera, *Almira,* before he was twenty. Handel is considered by many as the greatest composer the world has produced, and his fame was gained during his early life.

MENDELSSOHN was both brilliant and famous at ten years of age, and had given public concerts in Berlin and Paris. He began to compose music for the piano, violin and other instruments at ten, and published a volume of his productions at fifteen. He composed his *Midsummer Night's Dream* at eighteen and was the idol of all civilization while yet in his teens. He performed his famous oratorio, *Paulus,* at twenty-six.

GEORGE MORGAN, for many years organist at the Brooklyn Tabernacle, was a good pianist at five; he played the entire service in St. Nicholas' Church, Gloucester, England, at eight; performed in the Cathedral at twelve, and led the boys' choir in the same edifice from his fourteenth to his twentieth year.

What Some Young Men Have Done.

WEBER, the celebrated composer, began to publish his famous operas at thirteen, and was conductor of the opera at Breslau, and had gained a great reputation for his talents at the age of eighteen.

ROSSINI, the greatest lyrical composer of the present century, spent his boyhood studying the Italian and German masters. His *Tancredi,* which made such a wonderful sensation, appeared at twenty-three and his masterpiece, *Il Barbiere di Seviglia,* was composed before he was twenty-six.

HAYDN, the noted German composer, was born in great poverty; he became a member of the choir of St. Stephens, Vienna, at eight and was one of the leading musicians of his time while yet a young man.

THEODORE THOMAS, the eminent American musician, began to play the violin in public at ten, and had won a wide reputation as a musician and was leader of his orchestra, that has enjoyed such great popularity, at twenty-six.

RUBINSTEIN, the celebrated pianist, began to appear in public concerts at eight and from that time forward his career was attended by a constant ovation.

LISZT, whose reputation as a pianist is unexcelled, began to play the piano when three years of age. He was a student of music at six; he was starring through Russia with great

Manhood's Morning.

success at sixteen, and was professor in the
Strasburg Conservatory of music at twenty-
three.

GUSTAVE DORE, the celebrated French artist,
began to make sketches for the journals when
a mere boy; he showed remarkable ability while
in his teens. He exhibited his painting, *Battle of Alma,* when twenty-three, and quite a
number of his masterpieces before he was
twenty-six.

BENJAMIN WEST, the famous American
painter, began to paint pictures when six years
of age. He was not encouraged in the art by
his parents, but he made colors out of berries
and leaves, and brushes out of a cat's tail; and
with this crude outfit attracted great attention
by his skill. He painted a water-color picture
at nine, which he claimed in after life, that in
some respects, he never excelled. When his
great painting, *Christ Healing the Sick,* was
exhibited in the Royal Academy in London, this
little picture was hung beside it. In his six-
teenth year he painted one of his masterpieces,
Death of Socrates.

MILLAIS, the notable English painter, gained
the first prize at the Society of Arts when only
nine, and won the principal prizes at the Royal
Academy when only eleven. He had completed
his celebrated paintings, *The Widow's Mite*

What Some Young Men Have Done.

and the *Tribe of Benjamin Seizing the Daughters of Shiloh*, before he was eighteen.

MICHAEL ANGELO, one of the greatest painters, sculptors and architects that the world has produced, began to show remarkable skill at an early age, and his paintings while yet a young man brought forth a new era in the art. He carved his celebrated colossal statue of David at twenty-two.

RAPHAEL, the illustrious Italian artist, was an accomplished painter at fifteen and completed his famous painting, *The Espousals*, at twenty. He entered the Vatican at twenty-five, where some of his frescoes and other paintings remain as monuments to his remarkable genius.

BERNINI, the famous Italian sculptor, painter and architect, began early to use the chisel; he had completed his much admired group, *Apollo and Daphne*, and gained renown at eighteen.

DAVID LIVINGSTONE, the famous African explorer and medical missionary, was born poor and placed in a cotton factory to learn spinning at ten. He bought Ruddiman's *Rudiments of Latin* with his first week's wages, and sat up nights until midnight and later to study, and thus acquired a knowledge of several languages, botany and theology, and graduated in medicine, and was exploring the "Dark Continent" at twenty-three.

Manhood's Morning.

HENRY M. STANLEY was a teacher in an almshouse at thirteen, and had crossed the ocean as a sailor at fifteen. He had fought on both sides in the Civil War, traveled over a large portion of the globe, was a famous newspaper correspondent and was on his way to Africa to find Livingstone while yet in his twenties.

LORD MACAULAY acquired a brilliant reputation as a scholar and debater, and had won various prizes with his pen while in his teens. He early began to publish his writings, and his famous essay on Milton, "the learning, eloquence, patriotism, brilliancy of fancy, and generous enthusiasm" of which surprised and fascinated the public, appeared at twenty-five.

LORD LYTTON published his first work, *Falkland*, at twenty-two and he was famous while yet in his twenties.

BENJAMIN DISRAELI, the British author and statesman, began to write for the press when a youth and gave to the world his first novel, *Vivian Grey*, at twenty-two.

CHARLES DICKENS began to write for publication at a very early age. His *Sketches by Boz* appeared when he was twenty-four and his *Pickwick Papers* and *Oliver Twist* while he was yet in his twenties.

WILLIAM LLOYD GARRISON began to write articles for the press at seventeen and was editing the *Herald* at nineteen. It was the struggles of these boyhood days of Garrison to which Lowell alluded when he said :—

"In a small chamber, friendless and unseen,
Toiled o'er his types one poor unlearned young man;
 The place was dark, ungarnitured and mean;—
Yet there the freedom of a race began."

He was in jail for writing anti-slavery articles at twenty-five and was the victim of a mob in the streets of Boston for the same offence while yet in his twenties.

WENDELL PHILLIPS, the eminent statesman and orator, dedicated his life to the cause of justice and truth in his childhood. Referring to the matter just before he died, he said to a friend: "When I was a boy fourteen years of age I heard Dr. Lyman Beecher preach on the theme, 'You belong to God.' I went home, threw myself upon the floor in my room, with locked doors, and prayed, 'O God, I belong to Thee; take what is Thine own.' From that day to this it has been so. Whenever I have known a thing to be wrong, it has held no temptation. Whenever I have known a thing to be right, it has taken no courage to do it." Mr. Phillips was only twenty-six on that memorable occasion when he, amidst the intense excitement and threatening mob in Faneuil Hall, climbed upon the platform, and in answer to the unpatriotic and despotic speech of James Tricothic Austin, Attorney-General of Massachusetts, said, " * * * Sir, when I heard the gentleman lay down principles which place the murderers of Alton side by side with Otis and Hancock, with Quincy and Adams, I thought those pictured lips (pointing to the portraits in the hall) would have broken into voice to rebuke the recreant American—the slanderer of the dead! * * * For sentiments he has uttered, on soil consecrated by the prayers of the Puritans and the blood of patriots, the earth should have yawned and swallowed him up."

THEODORE PARKER, the eminent theologian and scholar, was teaching school at seventeen, and a few years later he was supporting himself in Harvard College by teaching private classes and schools, and applying his spare moments to the study of metaphysics, theology, Anglo-Saxon, Syriac, Arabic, Danish, Swedish, German, French, Spanish and modern Greek. He was one of the leading thinkers of the nation and editor of the *Scriptural Interpreter* at twenty-six.

JONATHAN PEREIRA, one of the most learned pharmacologists of any age, began his life-work when a boy and published a translation of the *London Pharmacopœia* at twenty.

DR. SAMUEL JOHNSON, the scholar, critic,

poet and lexicographer, was born in poverty and was frail in body, but kept a diary from his early childhood and in October, 1719, when he was ten years of age, he wrote in it the following; *"Desic tixe valedixi; sirenis istius cantibus surdam posthac auvem obversurus,"*—I HAVE BIDDEN FAREWELL TO SLOTH AND INTEND HENCEFORTH TO TURN A DEAF EAR TO THE STRAINS OF THAT SIREN. He was in the full tide of his literary career while in his twenties.

JOHN TYNDALL, the eminent scientist, chemist and scholar, was employed in a surveyor's office during his early boyhood. One day a fellow workman noticing his ability to learn advised him to devote his spare hours to study. The next morning John Tyndall, then not over twelve years of age, was out of bed and at his books before five o'clock, and for twelve years afterward he never swerved from the practice.

GOETHE, the illustrious German author, could write in Greek, Latin, French and other languages at nine. He composed his poem, *Joseph and His Brethren*, at twelve. His published writings began to appear while he was yet in his teens. His romance, *Sorrows of Young Werther*, was published before its author was twenty-five. It has been said of this work, "Perhaps there never was a fiction which so startled and enraptured the world; in Germany it became a people's book hawked about

96

the streets; it was the companion of Napoleon in Egypt, and in the Chinese Empire Charlotte and Werther were modelled in porcelain."

JOHN JACOB ASTOR, the famous millionaire, was born in Germany but had emigrated and was in business in New York at nineteen. He had accumulated two hundred thousand dollars, an immense fortune in those days, at twenty-six.

COMMODORE VANDERBILT was born poor but had established a ferry across the East River at seventeen, and at twenty-three had saved nine thousand dollars, a large sum at that time.

JAY GOULD was keeping books for a blacksmith at night to pay his way at school during the day, at fourteen; at fifteen he was working from six A. M. till ten P. M. in a store, and rising at three o'clock in the morning and studying surveying and mathematics for the three hours before business hours. He was surveyor and author before he was twenty-one; a tanner, a large lumber dealer, business man and capitalist before he was twenty-five.

STEPHEN GIRARD was a sailor, sea captain and successful merchant before he was twenty-six.

P. T. BARNUM, the celebrated showman, was clerking at thirteen; was in business at eighteen, editor of the *Herald of Freedom* at nineteen, and was making fifteen hundred dollars

What Some Young Men Have Done.

per week exhibiting Joyce Heth, nurse of General Washington, the "greatest show on earth," when he was twenty-four.

HORACE GREELEY, the founder of the *New York Tribune,* could read anything at four; had read the Bible through and could spell any word in the English language at six. He decided at eleven to be a printer and apprenticed himself at fourteen; was a publisher at twenty-two, and although his uncouth manner and ugliness were a great hindrance to his progress, he was famous as a literary genius while yet in his twenties.

HENRY WATTERSON, the noted writer and newspaper editor, had learned the printing business and was an editor at eighteen, and was one of the famous newspaper men of America at twenty-eight.

GEORGE W. CHILDS, the eminent American philanthropist, left home to seek his fortune and was in the United States navy at thirteen. He was born poor but he was rich in industry and perseverance, and was clerking in a Philadelphia book store for two and a half dollars a week and saving part of his income at fourteen. He displayed a remarkable aptitude for business and liberality even as a child, and had accumulated a fortune at twenty-five.

SOLOMON, "the wisest ruler that ever lived or ever will live," ascended the throne at eighteen. "The wisdom of God was in him to do judgment," and he began to build his great temple at twenty, and it was finished while he was yet in his twenties. Of the nineteen kings that followed the reign of Solomon the ages of seventeen, at the time they ascended the throne, are given. Of seventeen, sixteen were young men.

DAVID, the king, psalmist and sweet singer of Israel, had seven brothers older than himself, yet he was chosen in preference to them all to sit upon the throne. When he stood up to be anointed, he was a mere youth, "ruddy and withal of a beautiful countenance and goodly to look to." Although called from the tending of sheep to the throne of Israel at the age of twenty—too young to be president, senator, congressman, legislator, or even to vote in America—his reign furnishes the most brilliant example of elevated character in a ruler that the world has produced.

SAUL, the first king of Israel, and God's own anointed, was selected because he was a powerful and choice young man, and when he was seated upon the throne, from hearts that "God had touched" went forth the prayer, "God save the king" for the first time in human history.

MOSES, the lawgiver and sacred historian, was "exceeding fair" at a very early age and was learned in all the wisdom of the Egyptians and was mighty in words and in deeds while yet a young man.

JOSEPH was sold by his brethren to the Ishmaelites for twenty pieces of silver at seventeen. In the house of the Pharaohs he rapidly grew in wisdom and influence, and was "ruler over all the land" and Grand Vizier of Egypt while yet in his twenties.

SAMUEL, the prophet and judge, was clothed with an ephod and a mantle and served in the temple when a mere boy. When he stood before Eli, the High Priest, and foretold the doom that was to come upon him and his sons, he was only twenty. "All Israel, from Dan even to Beer-sheba, knew that Samuel was established to be a prophet," while he was yet a mere youth.

DANIEL, the prophet and courageous court minister of Babylon, began his life's work while a mere boy. By prudent conduct, personal honor and wisdom, he was made "ruler of the whole province of Babylon," and chief of the Governors over all the wise men of Babylon while yet a young man. When "he purposed in his heart that he would not defile himself with the portion of the king's meat, nor with the wine which he drank" he was only a child.

SAMSON, the judge and deliverer of Israel, showed his great physical strength and wisdom

100

in his boyhood. At twenty he killed the lion "as though it were a kid," and with the jaw-bone of an ass, he put forth his hand and slew a thousand men therewith, when he was twenty-one.

JOSIAH was appointed king of Judah at eight years of age. He began to seek the Lord at six-teen, and was actively engaged in purging the nation of idolatry at twenty.

JEREMIAH, the great prophet, began his sa-cred mission when a small boy. His plea for keeping silent was, "Ah, Lord God! behold I cannot speak, for I am a child." But the Lord put forth His hand and touched his mouth and he was a great prophet, "a defenced city and an iron pillar and brazen walls against the whole land," before he was ten years of age.

ELISHA was young in years when he be-came the prophet of Israel. He was plough-ing in the field near the road leading from Da-mascus to Horeb when the mantle of Elijah was placed upon his shoulders, and leaving his plow and kissing his father and mother fare-well, he at once began his great work.

SAUL OF TARSUS learned the trade of tent-making while a mere lad and, at thirteen, went to Jerusalem to prosecute his studies in the learning of the Jews and to study law under the great teacher, Gamaliel. It was to this period of his life, no doubt, that he referred

What Some Young Men Have Done.

when he said, "When I was a child I spake as a child, I understood as a child, I thought as a child, but when I became a man, I put away childish things." He was a faithful and zealous Pharisee, and while young in years distinguished himself as an able champion of his faith. He was converted and was a leader in Christian precepts and preaching while yet in his twenties.

SHADRACH, MESHACH AND ABED-NEGO, the three Hebrews who were cast into the fiery furnace because they would not fall down and worship the golden image which Nebuchadnezzar had set up in the Plains of Dura, were young men. With Daniel, they were "children in whom was no blemish, skillful in all wisdom and cunning in knowledge, and understanding science."

JOHN THE BAPTIST, as a child, grew and waxed strong and spent his boyhood in retirement, and when he began to preach in the wilderness he was a young man.

JOHN, the beloved disciple, was only twenty years old when called as an apostle.

JESUS CHRIST, the Incarnate Son of God, was about His Father's business at twelve. He "waxed strong in spirit and was filled with wisdom" while yet a child, and sat in the temple in the midst of the doctors both hearing them and asking them questions, astonishing

Manhood's Morning.

all by His questions and answers. He increased in wisdom and stature and in favor with God and man, and performed and finished His mission while yet young in years and in His physical prime. During His life He constantly complimented and honored youth. His disciples were perhaps all young men. His miracles and parables show a special devotion to young people. When He fed the five thousand He did not make use of the wise and strong, but took the five barley loaves and two small fishes from a boy. When He wished to teach who should be greatest in the kingdom of heaven, He did not point to His most faithful follower, but lifted an innocent and trustful child to illustrate the virtues which lead men to heavenly high places. The titles which are most full of sympathy and tenderness are those which reveal the youthfulness of our Saviour. He is the "Bright and Morning Star," the "Holy Child," the "Only-begotten Son," the "Dayspring," the "Lamb of God," the "Prince of Peace."

CHAPTER IV

Wild Oats and Other Weeds

Now as Jannes and Jambres * * . *Paul.*

"Our fathers to their graves have gone,
 Their strife is past—their triumphs won;
But sterner trials wait the race,
 Which rises in their honored place—
A moral warfare with the crime
 And folly of an evil time."—*Whittier.*

It looks very much as if existing tendencies were in the dead-line of vice.—*Josiah Strong.*

And at the town there is a fair kept, called Vanity-Fair: it is kept all the year long.—*John Bunyan.*

No sooner is a temple built to God, but the Devil builds a chapel hard by.—*Herbert.*

When a yung man beginz tu go down hil evrithing seams tu bee greezed fur the ockashun.—*Josh Billings.*

"The bird which is ensnared by one leg is as surely the prey of the fowler as if it were seized by both wings."

"He that spares vice wrongs virtue."

Better be unborn than untaught; for ignorance is the root of misfortune.—*Plato.*

CHAPTER IV.

WILD OATS AND OTHER WEEDS.

THE subject of morals is a serious and delicate study. To unfairly shade the moral character of an individual or any class of individuals is not only a gross injustice but it is slander. Be the facts what they may, questions which involve moral character should never be discussed, nor commented upon, except to commend and praise, unless some definite salutary end is to be achieved.

The truth should be scrupulously followed in all such discussions. A sacred responsibility always attends the publication of facts regarding adverse moral conditions. Parading and advertising sin and wickedness before the public often rivals, if it does not surpass in its demoralizing effects, the direct injury inflicted by their committal. Immoral gossip is of itself a loathsome disease and never a remedy. None should discuss the subject without earnestly praying

Manhood's Morning.

"Fair charity, be thou my guest
And be thy constant couch my breast."

I am not among those who believe that the young men of America are devoid of virtue and goodness. On the contrary, I know they furnish innumerable examples of manhood of the highest and noblest type. In every community may be found young men who are noble in heart and pure in character. They can be found in every postition in life. They may be poor in purse, brawny of muscle and ordinary of brain, but they are the salt of the earth and the light of the world; veritable temples in which dwell the attributes of divinity and the higher qualities of manly character.

The thirteen million young men of America, taken as a whole, represent inherent powers for development, somewhat latent though they may be, that are inexpressibly inspiring and full of promise. They are honest, industrious, patriotic and noble-hearted. They are in full sympathy with the principles of liberty, truth and justice. They are of honorable birth; they can boast of patriotic and virtuous ancestry. Their inherited and natural characteristics are an embodiment of those traits of manhood which insure national honor and which maintain with sacred loyalty the duties of citizenship.

It is an incontrovertible fact that the past

108

Wild Oats and Other Weeds.

has been marked by an improvement in morals.
Mankind is growing better. The standards to
which men must aspire are, however, constantly being raised. The world is improving and
demanding better men. The standards have
advanced more rapidly than men have. While
men have improved they are further from the
standards—from what they should be—than
ever before. While men were never so good as
now the imperative demand that they climb to
a still higher plane was never so great.

*It must be admitted that vice and evil habits
continue to rage in the land.* It must also be
admitted that young men are the chief trans-
gressors. From one border of our country
to the other, among the high and the low, the
cultured and the ignorant, the rich and the
poor, the prominent and the obscure; wherever young men abound, there come unmistak-
able evidences of a moral degeneracy deplorable in the extreme. Never in the history of
our nation were vice and immorality so power-
fully and systematically organized as they are
to-day. Wickedness revels and wallows in
moral filth and fatness and young men, legion
upon legion, are charmed and led astray by its
fascinations, and, filled with a wild passion for
pleasure, they sacrifice the flower of their manhood at its bidding, and worship at its shrine.
Indeed, personal and social impurity, vice,

evil habits, intemperance and morbid dissipation have become recognized characteristics of
the young men of the nation. In too many
homes may it be said

"The tones of every household voice
  Are grown more sad and deep,
And the sweet word—brother—wakes a wish
  To turn aside and weep."

There are few epithets more stigmatizing
than to say that a young fellow "has gone like
most young men." It means that he has gone
to the bad. To gain the reputation of being
"one of the boys" is little short of ill repute.
It is a sad fact that the experience of too many
of our boys and young men from their earli-
est career as such, is little else than a panorama
of vice and wickedness.

Those who have made a study of secret and
social sins are appalled at the terrible array of
facts which confronts them. This should not
be so. Because the time has come when a high
rating must be placed upon manhood. An inevitable result of advancing civilization has
been to bring the physical and moral natures
of men into close relations. As man progresses
in the upward scale an increasing demand is
made for the exercise of all his parts—muscle,
mind, talents, genius and heart—and the prob-

Wild Oats and Other Weeds.

lem of bringing all these attributes of his nature into harmonious action must not remain unsolved. When men gained a livelihood almost wholly by manual labor, physical strength was a chief virtue. But man's duties now consist of responsibility rather than labor, and call for powers of a higher and more complex nature than simple physical force.

Never were vice and wickedness so vitally antagonistic to success, prosperity and progress as they are to-day. Morals have become an economic question. Virtue to a remarkable degree has become a fundamental principle of our government. All genuine progress must be marked by the increase of moral cleanliness and the spread of social purity. Every young man who forsakes a high moral standard becomes less and less a part of the national greatness in the highest and best sense.

Many people seem to regard vice, evil habits and the various species of "wild oats" as simply morbid growths, like warts on the fingers or corns on the toes, and believe that some day they will mysteriously disappear never to be seen or felt again. Such delusions ruin more young men than war, pestilence and famine combined. Vice is the devil's weapon, and its mission is to ensnare, delude, blight and damn. When a young man acquires the habit of the smallest vice he opens the way for others.

Manhood's Morning.

No matter whether it be physical, mental, or moral, the contagion runs through the entire nature.

"Faults in the life breed errors in the brain,
And these, reciprocally, those again,
The mind and conduct mutually imprint,
And stamp their image in each other's mint."

Thus it is that evil habits and vices of all kinds are so closely related—always associated, acting and reacting upon each other—that it is impossible to tell where they begin, or just how much any single one insures or helps the work of ruin.

Irreverence is almost an universal vice among young men. A deplorable lack of reverence is shown for superiors and for sacred things, for parents and for the aged, for womanhood, for religion and for law and order. Perhaps of nothing else are young men so universally guilty. The coarse remark, the unkind ridicule and the cruel whisper is seldom suppressed or even rebuked. They find it so easy to sneer that they take to it naturally. Milton says: "A beardless cynic is the shame of nature," yet they can be found everywhere. Young men are more given to idle gossip, to defamation and to scandal than any other class. Says a recent writer: "Women are rapidly going out

112

of the gossiping business and men are taking their places." This assertion is too true. Young men are the most heartless gossipers in the world and by none is calumny prated with such merciless injustice. They originate more blighting and ruinous defamations of virtue and character, and feed the flames of scandal with more indifference and rancor, than all others combined. Filial affection and honor toward parenthood and a devout and manly reverence for religion and holy things are virtues sadly too rare. The tender and humane, the merciful and reverential in man are greatly in need of cultivation.

Reverence and respect for that which is higher and greater than we are, show the stamp of good breeding. The young man who fails to develop these virtues in his life robs himself of the most manly and elevating possession. Reverence toward parents, the aged, womanhood and God, gives to young men a nobility of character secured in no other way.

Vulgarity is a national curse. The habit of saying and doing vulgar things is a common vice. Vulgar yarns, stories and jokes, vulgar by-words and smutty phrases and off-color insinuations travel like wildfire among young men. Indeed masculine conversation is besmirched with these things. They find their way into the newspapers, dime novels and much of our cheap literature. Let a real smutty joke be unearthed within some focus of iniquity in New York City and it will climb the Alleghenies, travel through the Mississippi Valley and over the western plains and be hawked about the streets of San Francisco in less than a week. It is the debasing and polluting feature of the language. Thousands of young men think or talk little else.

Almost all knowledge imparted to boys concerning the sacred relations of the sexes, and of the transmitting forces of life is clothed in language as vulgar and obscene as ever echoed in the streets of Sodom. It flows like the breath from lip to lip, from men to boys, from boys to children until its blighting and damning voice is heard upon every side. As a consequence there is an indellible immoral taint to the imagination of almost every mind.

Vulgar pictures meet the gaze everywhere. Cigar and tobacco stores are panoramas of artistic lewdness. Advertisements of cheap theatrical performances cater to sensuality almost entirely. They are so made because the morbid tastes of young men are attracted by the carnality which they suggest.

No bait is more captivating to the average young man than a questionable picture, and cigarette manufacturers have, by offering such as prizes to purchasers of their goods, wrought an injury upon youthful minds only surpassed by the smoking of their vile and drugged concoctions of tobacco.

The naked bosom of the ballroom and dance hall and the padded legs in silken tights upon the stage, simply meet a popular demand for such things. Their influence upon the moral character of young men is such that the devil and all his angels might be challenged to produce something more alluring and vile in results.

It is not the nude, but the vulgar in nature and art that leads to defilement of mind and heart. A picture or statue does not have to be nude to be vulgar. Indeed, this has but little to do with it.

A British painter was criticised for exhibiting nude pictures upon the walls of the Royal Academy at each annual exhibition. In response to the criticism he exhibited, the following year, two pictures, one of which was remarkable for its purity, yet entirely nude, and the other a female figure entirely draped with the exception of one eye. In that one eye he depicted suggestions which he had always labored to avoid in other paintings, thus proving that vulgarity and sensuality are entirely distinct from genuine art and beauty. An artistic picture or piece of statuary may stand out in absolute nudeness and yet inspire pure and noble thoughts. When art is fashioned in vulgar curves and expressions, what would otherwise be proper, becomes an arrow laden with sensual poison ready to pierce the heart of any and all who will yield to the tempter. Art has a responsible and sacred mission in the cause of reverence, purity and virtue.

Profanity rages among young men. It is said that "profanity is our national sin," and that "America is the profanest nation in the world." These assertions are too true. Old men swear, young men swear, boys swear, children swear. Curses—deliberate and vile, cowardly and terrible, bloodcurdling and blasphemous—can be heard upon every side. There are legions of young men who cannot emphasize what they have to say unless they resort to oaths to do it. Profanity takes the place of adjectives, adverbs, interjections and exclamation points. The language of some persons is distorted almost beyond comprehension by oaths. When they are in society which is too decent to tolerate vile, blasphemous speech they are totally incapable of expressing their ideas.

The chronic swearer becomes constitutionally afflicted. The habit becomes second nature and an organic part of the language. Such victims always lament their fate. They despise the habit but they are its slaves. Profane language is the most execrable and vile that pol-

Wild Oats and Other Weeds.

lutes the tongue and of all men the victim of such a habit is one of the most pitiable.

Swearing is not only a useless but a stupid habit. It soon creates a poverty of expression and betrays a morbid and depraved mind. It tends to destroy refinement and culture and promote a coarse and brutal instinct. No matter how brilliant in mind or how generous in spirit a man may be, the habit of profanity will warp and contaminate his mind, and destroy the finer and nobler qualities of his character.

Vulgarity and profanity are twin vices. They co-operate in working injury. They are both mental habits and tend to destroy the very best part of man—his self-respect, his personal magnetism and his love for that which is virtuous and beautiful.

Tobacco is used by young men to a deplorable extent. Its use is not far from universal. Legions chew it, legions smoke it, legions use it in both ways. Tobacco is the *Youths-bane* of modern civilization. The cigarette fiend is legion.

About $750,000,000, are spent annually for tobacco in the United States. This vast sum is chewed and smoked up, and young men consume a large share of it. If this vast sum were turned into houses and furniture it would give to one thousand young men a fifteen hundred dollar house, furnished with five hundred dol-

117

lars' worth of furniture, every day in the year. In other words, it would handsomely supply one thousand newly married couples with a respectable house and home every morning.

According to the Report of the Commissioner of Internal Revenue for 1900, there were manufactured in the United States during that year, for home consumption, the enormous number of 3,258,716,305 cigarettes. Nearly all of these are smoked by young men. If these cigarettes were laid end to end in a row they would encircle the earth three times. It takes about ten minutes to smoke a cigarette, at which rate, to consume our annual out-put, it would keep busy, for ten hours every day in the year, no less than one hundred and forty-eight thousand men.

During the same year there were manufactured 6,176,596,421 cigars. It takes about fifteen minutes to smoke a cigar, at which rate, to consume the number manufactured, it would require four hundred and thirty thousand men, smoking ten hours per day, every day in the year.

But this is not all. There were manufactured during the same year 101,548,467 pounds of smoking tobacco. To smoke this quantity would require, smoking ten hours daily, about one and one-fourth million men.

The habit of smoking in our nation is equal

to nearly one and one-half million men smoking ten hours daily and fully one-half of this is done by young men.

There were used in the manufacture of the cigarettes 13,000,000 pounds of tobacco, and in the cigars 104,000,000 pounds of the weed. With this vast amount of nicotine poison were put immense quantities of opium, valerian, guiaic and other drugs, all intended to make the habit more fascinating and the effect more sedative and deceptive.

The annual production of manufactured "plug" and "fine-cut" was 185,353,411 pounds. There are at least one hundred chews in a pound of tobacco, and each chew will consume about one-half hour. At this rate it requires two and one-half million men, each chewing ten hours daily, to masticate the annual output.

The great army of tobacco consumers, supposing that each one is either chewing or smoking ten hours daily, Sunday included, may be calculated about as follows:

	MEN REQUIRED.
Smoking 3,258,716,305 Cigarettes	148,000
" 6,176,596,421 Cigars	430,000
" 101,548,476 lbs. Tobacco	1,225,000
Chewing 185,353,411 lbs. Tobacco	2,500,000
Men chewing or smoking 10 hours daily ..	4,303,000

This is equal to two-thirds of all the men

in the United States devoting three hours daily in using tobacco. This estimate is surely very conservative. What a tremendous power this subtle and destroying narcotic poison exercises over American manhood?

When we consider that nearly all the cigarettes, at least one-half of the cigars, and a large share of the smoking and chewing tobacco, are consumed by young men, the extent to which they indulge in tobacco is partly realized.

While many old men use it, yet nineteen-twentieths of them acquired the habit when young. At least one thousand boys and young men begin to use tobacco every day in the year. Many of them get their first lesson by picking up cigar stumps in the streets, cast away by Christians, and suck themselves sick. Others, to secure the weed, pick the pockets of their fathers, and, in seclusion, learn to smoke and chew like their elders. A whole legion, tempt-ed by vulgar and alluring prize pictures, spend their pennies for cigarettes, and treat their companions in imitation of the common custom among men. No vice so decoys its victims to habits of personal nastiness, deceit, dishonesty, licentiousness and profligacy.

While less money is spent for tobacco than for liquors, it is so much cheaper from a physiological standpoint, that the consumption of tobacco should be considered as vastly greater than that of liquors. Ten cents will purchase twenty cigarettes, from one to several cigars, and many chews of tobacco, while it will buy only two glasses of beer or one glass of wine or whiskey.

The annual product of tobacco in the United States is over 400,000,000 pounds. It contains from two to eight per cent. of nicotine, which is a deadly poison. One pound of tobacco contains poison sufficient to kill three hundred men if taken in a way to secure its full effects. If what is chewed and smoked were swallowed it would kill every man, woman and child three times a day. If young men consume one half of it they smoke and chew enough poison, if taken inwardly, to kill them five thousand times annually or, a fatal dose every two hours, were they not accustomed to its use, daily the year around.

Intemperance is common among young men. There is serious danger of America becoming a nation of drunkards. For forty years the per capita consumption of alcoholic liquors has rapidly increased. It is increasing at the present time. In many localities the man who don't drink more or less is the exception and not the rule. Especially is this true of young men. They are attracted to the barroom almost as easily as pigs are to the swill.

Manhood's Morning.

There are about 250,000 liquor and beer saloons in the United States, or one for every
fifty young men. The people annually consume
over over one hundred million gallons of strong
liquors and about one billion gallons of beer.
There are sixty drinks of liquor and about
sixteen drinks of beer in a gallon. This would
make six billion drinks of liquor and sixteen
billion glasses of beer, or twenty-two billion
drinks altogether, which find their way, every
year, down the throats of the American people.
It would seem that more than one-half of this
is drank by young men. This allows over
eleven hundred drinks annually to each young
man, or three drams every day in the year.
From time to time an effort has been made by
Christian Associations, and by those interested
in the subject of young men, to find out to
what extent they drink as compared with those
older in years. The result of all investigations
reveals the fact that overwhelmingly young
men compose the drinking class. Instead of
"old toper" we should say "young toper," as
the great majority of such appear to be young
men.

The following data were collected by reliable
persons under special instructions and show
what is going on all the time in almost every
populous section of our land. The figures are
not guess-work, but are actual counts made

upon the spot. In a city of 32,000 inhabitants 600 young men entered five of the prominent saloons in one hour. There are one hundred and thirty-five saloons in the city. In a city of 30,000 population 452 young men entered four saloons in two hours. In a large western city 478 persons were seen to enter a single saloon in one night and nearly all of them were young men. In another large city 236 young men went into a prominent saloon in one hour. In a town with 11,000 population 725 young men visited thirty-four of the fifty saloons of the city in one night. In an eastern manufacturing city, the Y. M. C. A. Secretary visited nineteen saloons during one evening and found 275 young men therein. Had he visited all the saloons of the city and found a proportionate number in each he would have found 6,000 young men in the saloons of the entire city.

In another eastern city, with a population of 130,000, during one Saturday evening, 355 young men entered five saloons in two hours. It was estimated that not less than 5,000 entered the one hundred saloons of the city during the same evening.

It is estimated that fully 4,000 young men enter a single saloon in one of our largest eastern cities daily. In San Francisco during one Sunday and Sunday night 15,933 young men were counted at base-ball, theatres, saloons and dens of iniquity, and the Sunday evening before 1892 young men attended all the churches of the city. In a city of 30,000 population there are 150 saloons and 1045 young men entered seven of them one Saturday night, and only 75 attended all the churches of the city next day. In a town of 7,000 inhabitants 130 young men entered three saloons in a single hour. In a city of 17,000 population more than one-third of all the young men in the city went into the drinking saloons in one hour during a Saturday night.

The above statistics, while not new, they can be verified at any time. Similar data have been collected under various auspices, and the unanimous result has been that North, South, East and West, wherever saloons exist, an almost universal habit of dissipation among young men is revealed.

The liquor bill of the nation has grown to be over *one billion dollars,* and the most of this money is hard earned cash from the pockets of young men who can ill afford to spend it. Nearly *two billion dollars* are annually spent for liquor and tobacco. Together they form the most gigantic and influential system of business enterprise the nation supports.

From one-third to one-half of this enormous sum is spent by young men. This means that

Wild Oats and Other Weeds.

they spend from $600,000,000 to $1,000,-
000,000 annually for that which inflicts a direct
and permanent injury. A very conservative
estimate would regard it fully one-seventh of
all they earn.

The use of tobacco and liquor is a wedded
vice. Young men drink because they use tobacco, and they use tobacco because they drink.
They forfeit their manhood and social standing, waste their health, time and money, disgrace their name and break the laws because
they use both. These habits destroy nerve
force, dwarf all the finer elements of manhood
and breed ignorance, filth and laziness. The
nicotine of tobacco, dissolved in the alcohol of
beer and whiskey, finds its way to the deepest
and innermost vitals. Thus commingled, they
force each other into action, the whole body
becomes poison-soaked and pickled, and only
the shadow of the original man is retained.
Within the vitals of the young men of America, these two elements are daily poisoning and
devitalizing untold millions of human beings
yet unborn, inflicting an inevitable curse upon
posterity, the result of which will be children
with debilitated nerves, impaired intellects, ab-
normal appetites and passions, and weakened
powers of will. The use of these two agents—
alcohol and tobacco—is inflicting upon the
young manhood of America, at the present

time, a greater curse than was ever wrought by any other agents upon any people in any age in human history. They challenge in their destructive effects the blackest and saddest records of either plague, famine, or war. To a remarkable degree they assist each other in human destruction. They are co-workers with the devil, and Satan himself, were he given universal dominion and power, could not devise two agents to operate more in harmony to dwarf, to degrade, to blight, to destroy, to kill and damn the men of the nation.

The vice of self-pollution is an existing curse. Those in a position to know pronounce it a common habit among young men. They are its chief and choice prey. In silence and in darkness, unheard and unseen, it spreads like a contagious disease, from one to many—from man to men and from boy to boys—until its influence is a national scourge, from which, alas! alas! too few escape. Unlike any other vice, it can be practiced without anyone but the guilty victim knowing it, until the effects of its ravages are written in the countenance.

It is impossible to know to what extent the habit prevails. It is enough to know that it is abroad in the land. Every student of moral and social conditions knows that it is a common evil, and that no vice is more strongly encouraged by passion. One writer of national

Wild Oats and Other Weeds.

reputation says: "The extent to which the habit is carried on is amazing." Another who has consulted a large number of prominent physicians upon the subject says: "Physicians of large practice can be found almost everywhere ready to testify that the habit is well nigh universal." That such statements can remain unchallenged is a disgraceful reproach, not only upon young manhood, but upon fatherhood and motherhood and every other force, be it Christian, heathen or pagan, that can wield an influence against this life and soul destroying sin. While there is no habit among the young to which parents and teachers should give more attention, yet there is none perhaps to which they give so little concern.

Licentiousness prevails among young men. The libertine, the leper and the moral rake are legion. The seducer of virtue struts in triumph upon every side. Our nation fairly swarms with young men who look upon woman as a fit subject for beastly indulgence. With one eye they will jealously guard their own kith and kindred, yet with the other eye they will watch for game upon which to satisfy their brutal natures and polluted appetites. It is a common belief that history is simply time revolving, and that at long intervals it repeats itself. It does seem 'that the wanton indulgences that have sent nations into disgraced oblivion were threatening American manhood. Greece, Venice and Rome, through prostitution, wantonness and libertinism, fell from eminence in civilization into darkness and ruin, and these vices are the menace that threatens America to-day.

The extent to which licentiousness is practiced is a question upon which opinions differ only in degree. All know that it is a prevalent and alarming evil. All conclusions must of necessity be largely guess-work. The vice is concentrated among women and diffused among men. Young men are its chief followers. Between twenty and thirty is the period in which men are most given to the habit. It is estimated that for every fallen woman there are from five to eight fallen men. The eminent Rev. B. D. DaCosta, D. D., of New York City, says: "If one wants to know the number of impure men in a community, all that is necessary is to find the number of impure women and multiply it by five." This rule will, no doubt, more than hold good.

The social evil in large cities is organized upon a business basis. Legions of young men flock into the great centres of population and find themselves surrounded by vicious influences which only the most determined qualities of character can resist. In many sections of the great West, prostitution, in an indirect way, is licensed, thus practically receiving the sanction of the law. Licentiousness—debasing, vile and doubly criminal—was the greatest curse connected with human slavery, and it still continues as a blighting and sinful outrage of the Southern States.

The police raids and exposures occasionally made in various large cities, while they show only the most flagrant transgressions, reveal a state of moral degeneracy very deplorable. It has been estimated that there are 40,000 prostitutes in New York City. This seems monstrous, yet the estimate is from reliable sources. More conservative observers place the number at 25,000. This evidently is entirely within the facts. Chicago, it is claimed, has 30,000. Pittsburg and other cities are not far behind.

A writer in *The Arena*, who is pastor of a church, in an article entitled, "The Social Evil in Philadelphia," says: "As many as five thousand women live among us by the sale of their bodies. I wish I might have confidence that the estimate is too high; but nearly six years of observation make me fear that the figures are much too low." This estimate includes simply what might be classed as "professionals" and does not embrace a "vast multitude" whose shame escapes the lawless bed-house and brothel. From the large cities, in an organized form, it finds its way into smaller cities and towns until its lecherous presence is everywhere. It has become insolent and bold and is condoned where, years ago, it would have been intolerable.

Licentiousness in the nation is not woman's but man's sin. Referring to the fallen women of New York City, Mr. Samuel C. Blackwell, a reliable authority says: "As a rule, each one of them was misled before she fell; cunning flattery, money, deceit, falsehood, possibly force led her to a fate she did not choose." Says Mrs. Dora Webb in a recent public address: "Immigrants arriving in New York City furnish 20,000 victims annually," and that "young girls are kidnapped, entrapped by deceptions, bought and sold for cash like slaves in the market of lust." And what is true of New York City is true the nation over. Mrs. Charlton Edholm, of Chicago, in a recent address in Baltimore, said: "I stand here in the presence of God to say that of the 230,000 erring girls in this land three-fourths of them have been snared and trapped, bought and sold."

Says Mr. J. B. Welty, a man of careful investigation: "To supply the demands of passion in men, one hundred families must give up a daughter apiece every day in the round year. What a draft is this on homes! What sin and shame and misery and heartaches and remorse and cruelty and murder and death and damnation this means!" How few of us re-

member and appreciate the words of the poet
who wrote:

> "O, wronged and scarred and stained with ill,
> Behold! thou art a woman still."

Men need to be taught that the social evil
is their affair. The degradation is their work.
Four-fifths of it is carried on by young men.
Social impurity the world over is man's power
against woman's weakness; man's cunning
against woman's credulity; man's willingness
to traduce against woman's nature to trust.
Too often it is his passions against her poverty,
and his subtle wile against her confiding
innocence. "Not one woman in a hundred
will seek her own shame." It is the unbridled
and fiendish passions of man that steeps our
nation in crimson crime, and not the seductive
charms of fallen women, as too many would
have us believe. Man is the artful designer
and aggressor, the seducer and adulterer and
woman is his victim.

Disgraced and fallen womanhood is not so
much a cause of licentiousness as it is a result
of it. Were Christ to again write with his
finger in the sands of earth what a multitude of
young men there are who could not look upon
the words! Were His example put in practice
in our nation to-day, how the tears of a redeem-

Manhood's Morning.

ed womanhood would fall at His feet; how
the mountains, dark corners and hiding places
would be filled with men! To what a vast
legion is the Seventh Commandment a dead
letter! What a horde of human brutes stand
ready to humiliate and disgrace the American
home! How little parenthood is honored; how
meanly sisterhood is prized; how contemptibly
virtue is esteemed? How villainy, while its
blood is hot with unholy lust, coos and caresses,
pleads and palavers, and when its mad passion
has made its conquests, how it skulks in triumph
while its victims, disgraced, ostracised and socially damned, are forced in silent remorse to
drink sorrow's bitterest dregs!

When homes have been pillaged of virtue
and fair daughters led astray, how deep is the
precipice over which they must fall! How
mammon's wild traders, organized for the purpose, gather them in and stamp their shattered
bodies with a price! How resistless is the
power that transforms filial affection into carnal mockery! How cruel is the tyranny which
demands that the sweet song of the sister become the silly strains of the siren and that the
sacred kiss for a lover become a medium of
lust upon the polluted lips of the leper! When
the sweet and beautiful souls of maidens have
become the black and blighted shadows of har-
lotry and scavengers in human flesh have stock-

132

ed their haunts of shame with such merchandise, what a legion of young men are, like brutes, only too willing to feed upon the offal!

The vice of gambling in many localities is common among young men. There is much more gambling going on than real good people suppose. Tens of thousands of young men are infatuated by it and its influence over them is enslaving in the extreme. Betting upon elections, prize fights, horse races, bicycle races, base ball, foot ball and other games, in the pool room and at the card table is a practice entirely too common.

Boys and young men are exceedingly credulous and they are easily infatuated by every kind of fake that offers much for little. Those whose earnings are small, and those with larger incomes, are all eager to swell their coffers. The temptation to resort to get-rich-quick schemes, in order to fill the pockets with cash, is keen and dazzling. The pathway of young men is literally deluged with captivating inducements to try their hands in schemes where luck, and not strict business methods is involved. Unprincipled sharpers reap a rich harvest from the hard earned savings of young men, and in return give only an opportunity to meditate upon their losses or plunge deeper into the entangling net of dishonesty and chance.

Ignorance is too common among young men.

Manhood's Morning.

By ignorance is meant a lack of that kind of knowledge which is essential to man's highest possibilities. There is an ignorance on account of which men do what is wrong, suffer disease and misfortune, and prematurely die. Ignorance is decay. "My people are destroyed for lack of knowledge," said the inspired writer. The young men of to-day lack this very kind of wisdom. Much of the wickedness and misery in the world is ignorance. The world is filled with tragedies that knowledge would have prevented. During times of peace competition and rivalry among men become intense, and to be intelligently equipped is the best guarantee of genuine success. Knowledge is power, safety and protection. A cultivated intellect, a trained reason, a disciplined will and educated faculties have become essential elements of citizenship.

It is necessary that man's education embrace a knowledge of not only physical and financial, but moral, social and spiritual things. To waste the intellectual powers upon insipid and nonelevating subjects entirely is the mistake of legions of young men. Newspapers which parade sensational news, accounts of prize-fights, police episodes, lapses of virtue and honor, sports of a low order, and which fill their pages with suggestive pictures and off-color slang and jokes, are the sort that are too generally popu-

lar. The pornographic titles of books sold for
five and ten cents at news-stands show the popular demand for literary trash.

Most young men have an acquired appetite
for morbid details and suggestive illustrations.
They read that which stirs the blood and
arouses the prejudices and passions. That
kind of knowledge which adds value to character and joy to life and which only a healthy and
pure mind can enjoy is discarded by multitudes
of young men. Such literature makes them
tired. The Bible is never opened by millions
of young men. The church is boycotted by
nearly as many. They do not read a verse of
scripture nor hear a sermon once a year. Only
a small per cent. are church members and a less
number are active in religious work. They do
not seem to consider moral and religious teachings within the scope of their needs. They are
not only ignorant, but oblivious of the needs
and activities of the moral and religious world.

At lectures and literary entertainments
young men are conspicuous by their absence.
Two of the most famous and entertaining orators in America, each recently delivered a lecture upon popular subjects—one lecture being
especially for young people—in one of our
largest cities, and although they were well advertised and delivered in a magnificent public
hall, in the heart of the city, not twenty young

men attended either; yet at the same hour over three thousand were attending theatres not ten squares away.

One of the most difficult problems with which our institutions of learning—literary, medical and law colleges, and even theological seminaries—are called upon to contend, consists in keeping under subjection the coarse animalism and unbridled sensual appetites of those whom they are trying to educate and train for the active and serious duties of life. Indulgent and well-meaning parents often use the college to reform their profligate and incorrigible sons. The effect has been to spread vice of an educated sort, and give to the cause of social iniquity, recruits, able and willing to champion its right to exist.

Lawlessness and crime are on the increase. Criminals of all kinds abound. Tramps, gamblers, bummers, loafers, dead-beats, confidence men, professional pick-pockets, thieves, highway robbers, burglars, murderers and petty criminals are not only numerous, but increasing in proportion more rapidly than the population. They are all largely composed of young men. Statistics tell us that the average criminal is twenty-six years and four months old, and that the reinforcements to the legions of law-breakers are almost entirely young in years. There are a vast army of tramps in the United States,

Wild Oats and Other Weeds.

wandering about without home or friends.
These men are tough, filthy, and, many of them,
infested with vermin. They sleep in the barns,
bushes and outhouses and beg from door to
door. An overwhelming majority of them are
young men.

A drove of professional tramps arrested by
the police of a certain city were described as
follows: "No tougher looking lot of men ever
passed through the door of the Central Sta-
tion than this collection of professional loafers.
They were all stout, able-bodied fellows, well
able to support themselves if they felt so inclined, and all of them between fifteen and thirty
years of age."

According to the last Census report there
were, 82,329 prisoners in the various penitentiaries and prisons of the United States, and
more than half of them were young men. There
were, at the same time, 7,386 persons in prison
charged with murder. Of this number 393
were women, but considerably more than one-
half were young men. Of the 45,233 persons
serving sentence in various penitentiaries only
1,791 were women, but young men composed a
large majority of the whole. During the past
ten years the number of female criminals has
decreased, but the number of males has very
markedly increased. During recent years murder has increased fivefold. The same Census

reports 14,846 children in the different reformatories, and of this number 11,535 were boys. The insane asylums contained 97,535 inmates; the almshouses, 73,045; the county jails, 19,535, and almost every institution in the land for defectives is crowded to the fullest capacity. While the majority of these unfortunates may not be young men, yet such conditions are more the result of wild oats sown by young men, who afterward become fathers, than all other causes combined.

Dr. J. W. Clokey, of Indiana, who has carefully studied this subject, says: "It is placing the figures inside the facts, rather than outside, to say that at any given time in the United States there are 150,000 convicts in its penitentiaries, prisons, jails and houses of refuge and correction." A good authority states that: "Not more than one-fifth of the active criminals are in prison at the same time." This would give our nation an enormous criminal population. Mr. Moody, in an address delivered in Philadelphia, said: "There are 750,000 persons in this country who belong to the criminal class, and statistics show that the number is increasing. In Massachusetts, in 1850, there was one criminal to every 800 of the population, in 1895 there was one criminal to every 225. More than half of the criminals are young men."

Wild Oats and Other Weeds.

*Indifference has become a national character-
istic of young men.* To the higher claims of
patriotism, morality, religion and humanity,
they show an apathy akin to deadness. There
is a disinterested lukewarmness among them,
both widespread and profound. This lack of
interest, on the part of young men, is one of
the saddest features of the new century upon
which we have entered.

Our military force, in the event of war, is
over ten million men, and should occasion demand it, they would, almost to the man, march
forth at the country's call. Our force in the
conflicts of peace is equally great. But it is
latent and unavailable. A heedless indifference
hangs like a pall over the young manhood of
the nation. Within its indolent embrace all are
made welcome. It is the enchanted ground of
the good and the enslaving refuge of the bad.
Under its composing influence men acquire the
habit of being nominally anything and radically
nothing; they cease to be either hot or cold,
good or bad; in nothing negative, in nothing
positive, but passive in everything. Under the
soft music of its lullaby, life lazily lounges in
the lap of time; the saints of God grow easy in
Zion; poverty and slavery, abject and cruel,
slumber in silence, the world, clothed in con-
formity, becomes wedded to indolence and sin.

Indifference, careless and unconcerned, is the

treason of the age. It cowardly looks on and blandly smirks while all that is vicious and wicked struts in insolent array. Swayed by its power, men cease to have any convictions in religion or principles in politics. Life's best motives are turned into the by-paths of policy and its most sacred issues are laid upon the altars of compromise.

Indifference is the consuming foe of manhood. It chooses ambition and industry as its prey and even robs genius of its power. It is the stagnant pool where settle the miasms of indolence and lust which poison and pollute the fountains of life. Under its shady bowers vice, crime and shame find shelter, feed and flourish. It strongly resembles—it must be—the unpardonable sin. It transforms the purest in mind into the vilest in thought and the noblest in character into the basest in action. It chills the enthusiasm, it dissipates the hopes and scatters the faith like the wind. It is deaf to duty, dumb to pity, and blind to care. It makes it possible to become dead in trespass and in sin. It saps the judgment, deadens the conscience and weakens the will. When indifference has gained the mastery the nobler impulses cease to direct, the moral nature atrophies and dies, the Holy Spirit is grieved away and man, in his moral and spiritual nature, becomes effeminate, powerless and undone.

CHAPTER V.

Some Reasons Why Young Men Go Wrong.

"Cast thyself down."—*The Devil.*

"Vice is a monster of so frightful mien
   As to be hateful needs but to be seen;
Yet seen too oft, familiar with her face,
   We first endure, then pity, then embrace."

"A child has a right to be born and not damned into the world."—*Bishop South.*

"He who teaches not his son a trade does as though he taught him to be a thief."

"Every man is the result of three factors—his ancestors, his surroundings and his individuality."

"Never since the world began has youth been so catered to; never has it been surrounded by so many open temptations; never so much flattered, and yet at the same time never have the reins of discipline been so relaxed."—*Amelia E. Barr.*

"It may be said with measurable truthfulness that half the art of Christian living consists in shunning temptation."—*J. G. Holland.*

"Hints shrewdly strown mightily disturb the spirit.
The sly suggestion toucheth nerves, and nerves contract the fronds.
And the sensitive mimosa of affection trembleth to its root."

CHAPTER V.

THE influences which shape the lives and mould the character of young men are varied and complex. Like everything else in nature, young men are an outgrowth of forces and circumstances for which they are not responsible and over which they can exercise but little control. Life does not begin at birth, but it runs back into ancestry. It is not bounded by the limitations of its own sphere, but it is a part of all the environments which surround it.

Many of the things which go to make up man are manufactured articles. The fact that so many young men are wayward and wild does not prove their guilt any more clearly than it proves that the forces which brought them into existence, and which have moulded them into what they are, have been faulty and corrupt.

Every one knows that the young manhood of America is surrounded upon every side by influences which strongly tend to weaken phys-

Manhood's Morning.

ical vigor, overthrow moral character and bring to naught the best energies and aims of life. "No man lives without jostling and being jostled; and in all ways he has to elbow himself through the world, giving and receiving offense."

The circumstances under which we are born and grow up have so much to do in moulding character and habits that it often happens that what the world sees of us contains only a fragment of our real selves. The powers which direct our footsteps are often so potent and so independent of our own design or intent that the lives we lead are extremely artificial. We instinctively imitate other people's manners and customs, we stumble over their mistakes and climb upon borrowed ladders, and too many lose their own individuality and live as a passive atom amidst a conglomerate whole.

At no time in human history, perhaps, were hindrances so numerous, seductive influences so subtle and man traps so broadcast and fascinating as now. So thickly strewn and so thoroughly organized are the besetments surrounding young men, that those who make a study of the subject·cannot feel other than surprised that uprightness and morality prevail to the extent they do.

A fair chance to live a useful, successful and peaceful life should be the common heritage of all. This chance is denied thousands of young men. It is made difficult for them to do right and easy to do wrong. They are exposed to influences—powerful and aggressive—which, from the beginning, conspire to lead them astray, thwart their success, impair their health, pervert their ideas, cripple their powers of reason, destroy their energy and ambition, mar their character, modify their sense of honor, destroy their lives and damn their souls. Inherited discrepancies, parental training, education, social customs, popular habits of life, and even much that apes religion, all more or less operate against the best interests of recruiting generations.

It is a fact that too few are well born. A frowning protest, during these modern times, stands at the threshold of parenthood, and too many of our race come into the world unbidden, unwanted and unblessed. When a child fails to receive the hallowed benediction of parental welcome and affection it is only half born. Young people marry who are criminally ignorant of the laws which govern the marriage relation. "There is no place where wisdom is so much needed or ignorance so disastrous as just here; yet we do not even think of studying it; the whole subject is left in midnight darkness."

Hereditary defects are accountable for much

of the evil we see about us. Inherited appetites and morbid passions prove a scourge among young men. There are many of the most debasing traits of mind and character which, though inherited, lie dormant until the hour when manhood begins to bloom, when, like hardy plants in a rich soil, they will grow and wax strong and crowd out all manly qualities and make ruin inevitable. Thousands of boys grow up, filling homes with joy and gladness and crowning parenthood with hopes and promise, only to find their manhood honeycombed by inherited sins, and their natures filled with passions and appetites which mow them down like grass.

The predisposition to crime and vicious habits, the appetite for alcohol and tobacco, the desire for licentious indulgences, and the whole category of morbid traits and temperaments, are inherited just as naturally as the color of the hair or eyes or the shape of the head or foot. Both science and experience prove that these things are not accidents.

Heredity closely follows inexorable laws, and the pivotal source between good and evil will never be understood until its laws are more closely studied; and genuine reform will never succeed until the lessons which these laws teach are put into practical operation. The warp of no fabric is more uniform than the threads of kinship which run down through the generations of mankind, from parent to child and to children's children, holding together, with consistent fidelity, the dominant peculiarities of body, mind and character.

It is inherited discrepancies, more than all else, that fill our homes with sickness and sadness, our jails with criminals, our almshouses with paupers, our asylums and charitable institutions with invalids, lunatics and imbeciles, and flood the country with vagabonds and tramps. Some years ago a reliable investigator (Mr. Dugdale, of the New York Prison Association,) traced the history of a certain family through seven generations, and, "Among 540 direct descendants, and 169 persons related by marriage or co-habitation, there were 280 paupers and 140 criminals of the worst sort; guilty of seven murders, of theft, highway robbery and nearly every other offense known in the calendar of crime. The estimated cost to the State of this family of criminals, paupers and drunkards was $1,308,000."

The celebrated John Cretien, with the taint of crime in his blood, was followed by three grandsons who committed murder, and nine great grandchildren, seven of whom died in prison. Of the remaining two, one was transported for highway robbery and the other was hanged. It is estimated by competent and care-

Manhood's Morning.

ful observers that from fifty to eighty per cent.
of crime and mental defects is due, in some
way, to heredity.

Immigration tends to lower the standards
of morality, and young men are the first to become influenced. While some of our best citizens have come to us from across the sea, yet a
constant stream of degenerates swarm from
other lands into America. It is an economic
policy of Europe to send to our shores its moral
and social debris. Nearly three-fourths of the
discharged Irish convicts find their way to
America. Immigration will not cease. Europe could send us 2,000,000 emigrants annually for a century and then increase her own already overcrowded population. Official reports
show that foreigners are three times as criminal
in their natures, and that they are five times
more apt to become paupers than American
born citizens.

Emigrants are composed largely of young
men. They come in contact with American
young men and the influence is vicious. The
influence of the foreign element in creating a
disrespect for religion, for law and order, and
in corrupting politics is constant and powerful.
The amalgamation between the races of the
earth, constantly going on in America, has no
parallel in human history. We are creating a
new people. The English, Irish, German,

148

Why Young Men Go Wrong.

French, Italian, Russian, Swede and Spanish;
the Protestant, Catholic, Jew and nondescript,
meet, commingle and marry, and out of the
amalgam is developing a new race. The nations of the earth are forfeiting their identity
upon American soil, and whether the reward
will be a fateful sacrifice or a rich and blessed
harvest the future alone can reveal.

Legions of young men are without a home.
There are in our nation two million young men
practically homeless. They are traveling as
salesmen, employes of railroads, steamboats,
vessels, traveling shows and other enterprises,
and as journeymen in all kinds of industry.
There are 250,000 saloons in the nation, and
from one to several young men can be found
behind the bar of almost every one. All of
these vocations require slavish devotion and
long hours of service and most of them operate
seven days in the week, giving no time for recreation or mental development, and no chance
to gain the elevating and moral influence of
home life. Their bread and butter come
through a continual plod. Day in and day out,
with no relief, they sacrifice comfort, lose sleep
and waste the best years of life in serving the
exacting demands of organized and incorporated greed and avarice. Their spare hours
and surplus dollars are boldly sought by an
endless variety of dissipations over which

149

the devil holds almost an absolute monopoly.

Not only are a vast multitude without a home, but the home training of as great a number is the opposite of what it should be. A New York Supreme Court Judge a few years ago said: "There is a large class of the population of New York and Brooklyn who just live, and to whom the rearing of two or more children means inevitably, a boy for the penitentiary and a girl for the brothel." A conservative estimate places the number of boys in Chicago without a home, or with a home worse than none, at ten thousand. Other large cities furnish their quota. The influence of such a prostitution of child-life, from every standpoint, is demoralizing beyond measure. A prominent Judge of Chicago says: "Most of these boys will turn out to be thieves and criminals. Each one of them forms a nucleus for a history of crime." Thus do legions of boys grow into manhood without knowing anything but poverty and squalor, and caring for nothing but depravity and dissipation.

Parents and well meaning people deplore the great temptations to which young men are exposed. Yet how few think to teach their boys to hate, and train them to overcome these things? They try to lubricate the pathway over which their sons must pass with a superabundance of kindness and sympathy, and forget that success, and usefulness, and virtue, and honor, and heaven and all other good things grow high and must be climbed after, and that the smoother the way is made the more apt young men are to slip and fall and miss the goal. The young should be taught to face and grapple with difficulties, as they are the stepping-stones to success; to endure trials, as they are the rounds in the ladder to heaven. They must learn that self-confidence and unaided efforts are necessary in climbing the rugged heights in life's highway.

Young men are not properly appreciated. They are not given a fair chance. This is true in a hundred ways. Responsibilities and opportunities unquestionably make men. When these things are withheld men fail to reach their full development in both body and mind.

The first desire that enters the mind of a new-born babe, regarding life, is to be a man. Becoming such is entirely natural. Its consummation is the highest achievement which finite conditions allow. It is a crime against humanity when any impediment is permitted to abridge the perfecting of manhood. Yet how often do we see, on account of errors in training, men whose whole natures are dwarfed; babies in pantaloons—petted, pampered and spoiled—wilful, cross and peevish—five and six feet tall—ten, twenty, thirty, forty years old—saucy, dirty mouthed and indolent. Such individuals, and every generation furnishes a crop, cannot be expected to do more than drift with the wind, tide and crowd, no matter in what direction they may be impelled.

The old are not always friends to the young. It is a difficult thing for those who have grown old to be in full sympathy with, and heartily encourage, their juniors. The man who gracefully welcomes his young rival with: "You must increase, but I must decrease," shows a rare martyrdom. A frog has no regard for a tadpole, having ceased to be one himself, and most men are similarly constituted. Old men, as a rule, distrust the capabilities, opinions and methods of young men.

But few children receive from their fathers the benefits of a wholesome discipline and training in ordinary business affairs. The wealth and wealth producing interests of America are, largely in the hands of men who have passed the prime of life. These men represent the past rather than the present, or rapidly unfolding future. It is too often the case that when a man dies, his children, for the first time, obtain an insight into the details of his business. Much of the inherited wealth, in consequence, proves an injury instead of a blessing. The eagle stirs her nest, bears her young upon her wings and teaches them to fly; mother goose gives her goslings swimming lessons in the nearest puddle, but thousands of young men are required to enter upon their life's work, and fail and go astray, because selfish and jealous greed, and not the Golden Rule, has been their school-master.

Multitudes of young men are led astray by evil companionships. Boys are taught profanity and vulgarity, taught to smoke and drink, taught personal defilement and licentiousness at a very early age. A blunt but most excellent man who spent his life among young men said: "The average boy of twelve is ruined." Thousands are dosed during infancy with soothing syrup, paregoric and other opiates and alcoholics, thus forever perverting their appetites. Vulgarity and obscenity circulate in the streets and among school children, and wherever boys and young men crowd together these things, as a rule, are freely indulged. Boys form bad habits and practice vice, indeed are often enslaved, before they know that such things are injurious and wrong.

Much of the literature of the present day is a curse to young men. Vulgarly illustrated periodicals and immoral fiction do incalculable harm. The great metropolitan daily newspapers keep up a constant panorama of crime, murder, conjugal lapses, prize fights and sensational exaggerations. The Sunday newspaper is the worst of all, and it is more read by young men than any week-day issue. The Sunday newspaper is the Church's worst enemy. Many of those published seem to know no propriety except what the law demands. Such literature destroys the finer qualities of the mind, and creates morbid imaginations which almost inevitably lead to immoral habits.

The New York Society for the Suppression of vice during a single year seized 63,139 pounds of obscene books, 836,096 obscene pictures, 1,577,441 circulars, songs, etc., and 32,-883 papers, and arrested over 2,000 persons for being engaged therein. The names and addresses of 1,102,620 persons were seized. Dealers in this class of literature use every means to get the names of boys and young men, and the business they do is tremendous. Says Mr. Anthony Comstock: "The degrading of the youth of this nation by the sickening details of loathsome crimes, the horrors of blood and thunder stories, the dime and half-dime novel and paper, and the foul oozings of defiled minds in many weekly papers, to say nothing of the nameless books and papers, is one of the highest crimes that can be committed against the future of this nation. These brutal assaults upon the native innocence of youth and children are laying burdens upon the rising generation which will be grievous to the future."

"A perpetual assault is made upon the citadel of thought. Secret hours are spent dreaming over the story of vice and crime. The receptive mind of youth drinks in sensational, foul and criminal story with an avidity that is fearful to contemplate. To those who have seen the results of these worse than sting of asps, no surprise is felt, when in after years is heard the moan of the aged person praying to be delivered from the sins of his youth."

The millions of quack medicine pamphlets distributed by "Private Disease" and "Lost Manhood" charlatans, inflict upon the minds of young men an exceedingly vile impression. They often create imaginary diseases similar to those they are advertised to cure. There are many books written upon immoral subjects, ostensibly to teach moral lessons, but most of them have been written simply to sell. Nearly all of them are to young men. Some of these books are most excellent but others are highly injurious. It is almost impossible to profitably moralize upon immoral subjects. "It is only in exceptional natures that familiarity with vice increases the horror of it." It is impossible to build up a chaste and manly character by parading sensuality, even in pious language under sanctimonious headlines. Rot is rot, and it is never more rotten than when it is sandwiched between religious quotations and antiquated poetry.

Manhood's Morning.

The discussion of the mysteries of sex, and of the transmission of life are subjects which, though important and sacred, have polluted more minds than any other one thing. Knowledge of these matters comes to ninety-nine boys in a hundred clothed in language as low and vile as the most depraved carnality can conceive. It would seem that the entire subject of sex and human biology has been handed over to the powers of evil to lead boys and young men astray. The influence of morbid teachings is blighting to the minds of the young and, in consequence, thousands are not allowed to indulge an unmolested chaste thought nor experience an untainted joy.

Parents are criminally guilty in neglecting to instruct children regarding these matters. Every father and mother should take their children into their confidence, and at a proper age, reveal to them the mysteries of sex, and the physiological laws pertaining thereto. They should not wait until it is too late, but do it early. This would prevent morbid curiosity, and give to a knowledge of these subjects the force of chastity and sacredness. I wish to here solemnly declare that if parents would intelligently and thoroughly do their duty regarding this matter a revolution in morals would ensue. When will boys and young men cease to learn of these things through channels which flow to destruction and in language that savors of the pit?

One of the most hopeful developments of modern literature is the advent of books that impart proper knowledge to the young upon subjects pertaining to sex. Among the best of these for young men are, "What a Young Boy Ought to Know", and "What a Young Man Ought to Know", and "What a Young Husband Ought to Know," all from the pen of Rev. Sylvanus Stall, D. D. These books are clean and instructive, free from insipid advice and should be read by every boy and young man.

Modern business methods and the means of livelihood are becoming more and more antagonistic to the success of new recruits. Those who are compelled to begin life without some special talent, a good supply of inherited wealth, or influential friends, are finding it extremely difficult to gain a foothold within the threshold of success. That desirable goal called success in life is to be gained only by a few. As with political offices, there is not enough of any business or calling to go around. The great mass of young men must be doomed to disappointment.

The road to success is literally crowded with giants, compared with whom average young men are as grasshoppers, and these kings and princes, monopolists and demagogues of trade are only too willing to deal vengeance upon any and all new accessions to their ranks. There may be "room on top" but the fellows who are already there do not think so, and those who undertake to rival them in achievement are apt to find not only a vigorous but crushing opposition awaiting them. One of the leading business men of America has said that "real good chances, except to a very limited few, are a thing of the past." It is the inevitable fate of most young men to wrestle with poverty and misfortune as a life-long struggle.

The fact that it is becoming more intensely difficult for men to earn an honest and respectable living is a most potent source of evil. A young man cannot serve God, his fellow man, nor himself, unless he has useful employment for his hands and mind. When Christ was upon earth he always fed the hungry before he began to preach to them, but the practical side of His religion has been greatly neglected.

There are, during seasons of business depression, hundreds of thousands of young men in our land who are either unable to find work of any kind, or must accept such employment as exercises only the crude and primitive powers of mind and muscle, leaving the talents and intellect indolent or idle. An enormous number of young men are little more than industrial vagrants, unwillingly made so by vicious systems of industry over which they exercise no control. Eighty per cent. of those who go into business fail, not so much because there is no room, as from the fact that the room is monopolized by the favored few. Competition and rivalry have become so intense that new ventures find it not simply difficult, but impossible to succeed. The veteran and the professional in any business or avocation know that only a few engaged therein can find a profitable basis. The great majority of those engaged in business must keep up a constant struggle to make ends meet. This strain to gain a livelihood falls more heavily upon young men than any other class. They are the greatest losers in lapses of trade and industry. A pronounced season of business depression proves a tremendous force in demoralizing morals and character. At such times young men conceive warped ideas concerning honesty, politics, religion and morality. They at such times are surplus stock. They become poverty stricken and their ambition, industry and talents are a glut in the market. They become humiliated to beggary before the power of capital. They are veritable slaves, and must accept the crumbs that fall from the table of business. "It is almost as depressing to beg for work as it is to beg for bread," and thousands of young men, the very cream of American

Manhood's Morning.

manhood, are constantly hunting a job. Nearly all young men begin life by seeking employment. Pre-eminently they are the wage earners of the nation. They are dependent upon others almost entirely, and in return have nothing to give but their services. Thomas Carlyle said: "A man willing to work and unable to find it, is perhaps the saddest sight that fortune's inequality exhibits under the sun." Nothing is more crushing than enforced idleness, thwarted ambition and unavoidable poverty.

Young men find every foot of land taken, owned and occupied; every business overrun, and every department of industry crowded to overflowing. And those who occupy and monopolize the activities of the world are holding on, and grasping, saving and hoarding, and many of them denying themselves and living poor for the sake of dying rich.

For every vacancy there are many applicants, and it is nothing unusual for several hundred young men to answer the same advertisement for help. This condition of affairs causes legions of young men to resort to questionable and compromising employment in order to secure clothing, food and shelter. It exposes them to a multitude of snares which they would otherwise escape. They abandon society; they cease to go to church; they avoid matrimony and become clandestine in habits, and, with morbid ideas of life and of duty, they become permanently unstable and shiftless.

Labor-saving machinery often operates against handicraft. New inventions are constantly supplanting labor. Improvements in labor-saving machinery render one man or boy capable of doing the work of two, twenty, and, in one or two instances, two hundred. The invention of the knitting machine affected fifty thousand people in England for two generations. The invention of the cotton-gin revolutionized the labor of the South, as it does the work of a legion of hands. The reaper and binder, while it was a potent factor in developing the West, proved a great annoyance to the working classes, thousands of whom depended upon the harvest fields as a source of employment.

With labor-saving machinery come new methods of doing business, the whole trend of which is to dispense with labor. Everything is being done on a large scale. The old method of beginning in a small way and working to the front has become almost obsolete. A beginner cannot rival those who already occupy the field. It don't pay to do business any longer on a small scale. A small manufacturer cannot make shoes, or cloth, or furniture for what a large manufacturer can afford to sell these things. "It costs seventy-five cents per bushel to grow wheat in a small way, but a large wheat grower can land it in the market at a cost of forty-five cents per bushel." When wheat sells for sixty cents per bushel, the large farmer makes fifteen cents per bushel, and his poor neighbor loses fifteen cents. The old established and gigantic business concern can buy goods for less money than the beginner, handle a large volume for what it costs to handle a small amount, sell for a less profit, secure advantages by having ready cash in abundance, secure better rates of transportation, keep a larger and better variety and be more liberal in every way in accommodating customers. Indeed everything bows to the power of money, and the modern giants in the realms of manufacture and trade are bound to be monopolists whether they so desire or not.

The concentration of wealth, as it exists in America at the present time, is an extremely discouraging condition to young men. There is a certain commendable pride and ambition forming an essential nucleus to every successful life, which if crushed, or destroyed, makes failure almost inevitable. When a young man stands at the threshold of his career and realizes that the wealth of the nation is gleaned and garnered, that his life must be one continual plod, and that his only reward will simply be the ability to keep soul and body together, a tremendous conquest for evil is wrought unless his manhood contains far better metal than the average.

I have said in a former chapter that the best thing that can come to a young man is to be thrown out into the world. This is true. Young men need such exercise to develop the powers of their manhood. As a rule they are better off if they start with nothing, but the chance to succeed must be kept open to them. It is only when poverty is a doom that it is to be feared. When poverty becomes the inevitable fate of young men they are no longer free, but slaves. That which we call liberty and freedom only exposes them to temptations and privileges which lead to ruin.

The total valuation of the real and personal property of the United States has increased enormously during the recent years and at present is not far from one hundred billion dollars. One hundred men own one-twentieth of this enormous sum. Forty thousand men own one-half of it. One million men own three-fourths of it. This means that seventy-five million of our people are worth about $25,000,-000,000, or only a little over $300 each.

There are over 13,000,000 families in the nation and one-half of them are not worth $200 each, or less than $40 for each individual.

Manhood's Morning.

This means that one-half of our population—
over 38,000,000 people—are not worth enough
to keep them in food and clothing through a
single winter.   They are poverty stricken.
These figures prove that a majority of the
young men of the nation start out practically
without a dollar.   They have neither money,
friends nor visible opportunity.   They are, too
many of them, tradeless, uneducated and un-
equal to meet the conditions required of them.
They find themselves a drug in the labor market.   Were they transformed into merchandise
their money value would be shamefully small.
Put up at auction, the average young man
would not bring as much as a good horse.
They in no way compare in money value with
the slaves of the South forty years ago.   The
moral effect of these conditions is withering,
and blighting, and deplorable beyond concep-
tion.

There are hundreds of thousands of young
men leading profligate and immoral lives because an infamous system, embracing business, commerce, industry and finance denies
them the opportunity of earning an honest and
respectable living.   They would become contributing and valuable citizens, faithful and lov-
ing husbands and fathers; they would establish
homes, build houses and add wealth and character to the nation were they given a chance.

Why Young Men Go Wrong.

But the wealth of the nation and the power which it possesses have conspired against them. Capital makes its own laws and dictates its own terms. It demands all the profits and the unconditional surrender of all its antagonists. The love of money and selfish greed have become master passions. Money makes monopoly possible and monopoly is almost always mammon-wild and heartless, and when it is, those who serve it must cower at its feet and be unto its storehouse as beggars and unto its authority as common slaves.

Another obstacle to the success of young men is the fact that during the past few years women have fairly swarmed into every department of human activity. They form, by far, the most formidable rival against which the young manhood of the nation is forced to contend. Women are the "better half," not only in the home, but in the store, the factory, the counting room and even on the platform and in the literary sanctum. Much is written and said about the demoralizing effects of the cheap labor of foreigners; the labor of women is more than simply cheap—*it is cheap and it is good.*

There are at present, especially in cities, almost as many women as men earning a livelihood. Many of them are doing what men should be doing. This condition gives to the idleness of young men a sad and hopeless phase.

Manhood's Morning.

Nearly one-half of the money that passes over the counters of the legitimate business houses of our large cities and towns is handled by women. Man is hopelessly her inferior as a rival in clerical work and persistent service. Women are more economical, more attractive, quicker of perception, more accurate, rapid, industrious and loyal than men. Their eyes are keener, their brain clearer and their fingers more nimble, and they are instinctively more adroit. They can do more work, and better work, for less pay, than men, and in many positions are much more acceptable.

Man can never cope with woman as a rival. Women are more subordinate and have less selfish interests than men. They apply themselves more closely to the work in hand, and, as a rule, are less meddlesome. They neither drink, smoke nor loaf, and they almost never prove dishonest.

Women, as a rule, make a more thorough preparation for a chosen pursuit than do men. Technical colleges and training schools for women are rapidly on the increase, and girls by the legion, are preparing themselves for every possible legitimate vocation. Their services are being sought in preference to those of the sterner sex. Young men are in consequence being driven hither and thither and the moral effect is worthy of the most serious concern.

Why Young Men Go Wrong.

Women are capturing some of the most desirable vocations almost en masse. Teaching, for instance, is rapidly passing into the hands of women. There are about 450,000 teachers in our nation, and already two-thirds of them are women. In Rhode Island, Massachusetts and New Jersey over 90 per cent. of teachers are women; in New York 85 per cent. In the sectional schools of Philadelphia there are 3,375 women teachers and only 216 men, and in New York City there are 19,013 women and only 1,411 men teachers. At the present rate of increase of the one and decrease of the other, unless a reaction occurs, male teachers will finally be a thing of the past.

It is estimated that there are over 40,000 type-writers and stenographers in New York City, and the great majority of them are women. A parallel statement would apply to the entire nation.

The increase of women wage-earners, from 1880 to 1890, was remarkable and the number continues to rapidly grow. During the above ten years women musicians and music teachers increased from 5,753 to 34,519; artists and teachers of art, from 412 to 10,810; actresses, from 692 to 3,949; bookkeepers, clerks and copyists, from 8,011 to 92,825; journalists, from 35 to 888; physicians, from 527 to 4,555; lawyers, from 5 to 208, and clergywomen, from

167

67 to 1,235. Not many years ago only a few occupations were open to women, now the field is practically theirs.

Not only has woman established herself as an industrial and business factor, but she is being felt in politics. Law-makers are beginning to yield to her demands for recognition and justice. "Equal pay for equal services, regardless of sex," is finding its way into political platforms, and, in some States, women are beginning to vote. She is doing it so willingly and well—and remains a woman still—that it is only a question of time when all barriers to her highest achievements and broadest activities will vanish. She will soon become a freeborn citizen and enjoy all its privileges. "Woman's sphere" will cease to have a limit. Unless young men reform, and bestir themselves, and redeem their wonted dominion, and marry their rivals, they will find themselves supplanted and ostracised from the realm of progressive enterprise.

Politics does much to demoralize the nobler traits of young manhood. Next to religion, politics is the most sacred subject that men are called upon to consider, but it has become corrupt and debauched. A United States Senator has said: "The Decalogue and the Golden Rule have no place in a political campaign." Men do in political matters themselves, and condone in others, what would be high crime in any other phase of action. The right to vote should awaken a profound sense of duty. But it does not. Politics has become the common resort of unprincipled and selfish men. In no other realm are corrupt methods and subtle treachery so effective. It furnishes a level where money and marketable manhood meet, and where fame and power can be bought with a price.

> "Strange dance! 'Tis free to rank and Rags;
> Here no distinction matters;
> Here Riches shakes its money bags,
> And Poverty its tatters."

It has been stated that no less than 85,000 men have either directly or indirectly sold their votes at an election in New York City. In every locality the "floaters" for sale completely handicap those who reverence and hold sacred the ballot box. Says a prominent American citizen: "Bribery and political corruption have become a portentious evil menacing the very foundations of our free institutions." The intimidation in politics is such that it requires almost as much courage to withstand a political campaign, by voting as one pleases, as it did thirty years ago to shoulder a musket and enter the conflict for freedom. Statesmanship has degenerated into bossism, and patriotism into partyism.

The realm of politics is so corrupt and unsavory that clean, self-respecting men are disposed to avoid it. Scheming demagogues have almost a monopoly fighting each other. It is too often the case that the more worthy and circumspect a man is the less influence, politically, he has. About all the influence which conscience and ·convictions exercise at the ballot box is to act simply as a balance wheel to keep the whole machine from utter ruin.

Nearly one million young men arrive at their majority each year, and at each presidential election over three million vote for the first time. More than any other class, they are sought, importuned, coaxed, deceived, lied to, elbowed, bribed and bulldozed.

Thus schooled, young men conclude that politics is a prize game; that popular government is a farce and that all there is in it is what can be got out of it. Thousands dismiss the principles involved from their minds entirely, and become as straws, leaning toward that party which makes the biggest display and which has the best prospects of success.

The church and other organized religious forces fail in their duty toward young men. The fact that young men are not being brought into the church and under moral influences is

apparent everywhere. In many places the
church is almost a complete failure. Yet religious people are in earnest. Never was the
church more active than now. In every department of Christian work a special effort has
been made to reach young men. To none has
philanthropy been more liberal, for none have
prayers been more fervent. The results have
not, however, been encouraging.

When we remember that most of the solid
character and moral worth, with which society
is blessed, is inherited rather than acquired;
when we learn how few—extremely few—
young men who start wrong ever reform and
become earnest, useful Christians, we must admit that the influence of religious organizations
is deplorably slight. Religion of the convicting
quality and converting quantity seems to be
wanting. We sing "Ninety and Nine" to *one*
sheep, while the *"ninety and nine"* are out "on
the desert bare." There is a great lack of practical force and spiritual power somewhere.

The work of religion is greater than the
work of science, of education or of culture,
greater than reforms or revolutions, than politics or political parties, than the pen or the
press. Its work is greater than all of these
things together. Its mission is to uplift and
save the world.

Religious institutions have become too much

engrossed in their own internal affairs. They dress parade, but seldom fight. They try to resave the saved rather than the lost; to make people believe exactly rather than trust implicitly. They spend their energy in the endeavor to make the good better and the better perfect; in salting the salt; in directing the way to their own pilgrims, leaving the lost sheep, for whom Christ died, to shift for themselves. The elder brother, the upright son, who has saved his money and who pays high pew rent, is feasted upon fatted calf, while the unfortunate prodigal is allowed to feed upon husks and spiritually starve.

There are several million young men in America who never hear the gospel preached. What little they learn of the subject of religion is gained by coming in contact with professing Christians. What they see and hear is so commonplace and disappointing that they relieve their minds of the subject entirely. When religion ceases to be aggressive, enthusiastic and in living earnest, young men, at least, forget that it has any special claims upon them.

Many good people imagine that pure, genuine, unadulterated gospel truth is not just the thing for young men, and a tremendous effort is made to make religion attractive, entertaining and even amusing in order to attract them. Addresses and religious meetings for young men are expected to possess at least three features,—they must be "spicy, entertaining and short." When.young men become Christians they are too often made into hothouse plants instead of shining lights; they are burdened with advice instead of work; they are not accepted as soundly converted until they have been well trained in the doctrines of some particular creed.

As a rule young men have planted, deep within them, an exalted reverence for sacred and religious things. They need nothing so much as gospel truth and Christian consistency among those with whom they do business and associate. They should come in contact with these things, not simply on Sunday, but seven days in the week.

During recent years there has been a wellmarked tendency for mankind to divide into widely separated classes. Evil always follows such a condition. Not only have wealth and avarice become organized, but selfishness and pride, as well. The rich and the poor, the strong and the weak, the fortunate and the unfortunate, the learned and the ignorant are inclined to stand apart and grow more exclusive. These conditions make vividly conspicuous everywhere man's inhumanity to man. A warfare, constant and relentless, exists, in some form, between these extremes. The fortunate

Manhood's Morning.

preach contentment to the unfortunate, and the less favored preach the Golden Rule in return, and both detest the precepts of the other. Class distinction, wrought out of human experiences, has been the curse of civilization. It is the apparent doom of Europe to-day. It is the underlying basis of most of the struggles in our own land.

> "O! Why should the strong oppress the weak
> Till the latter goes to the wall?
> On this earth of ours, with its thorns and flowers,
> There is room enough for all."

The lines of conflict between the high and the low constantly grow more apparent. Should we discover that such conditions are compatible with the spirit of liberty, it would only prove that our boasted liberty is a misnomer.

Widely separated class distinctions, in any phase of life, are to be deplored, because such conditions always handicap genuine progress. Mankind is a common brotherhood, and conditions and systems which bring all classes of people together in harmony must prevail. Science, Education and Social Agencies have become active factors in the world's progress. New conditions confront us. A new era of progress is close at hand. Superficial and narrow views are no longer effective. The best welfare of all, and not selfish factions—too long the American octopus—must prevail.

Why Young Men Go Wrong.

Scientific workers were never so closely allied to progress, health and happiness as at present. That man is his brother's keeper has become a scientific fact. Scientists have become the kings of earth. Knowledge of health, sanitary matters, hygiene and thousands of other economic branches, are forcing a new era. Science is proving that vice is an organic disease, reaching back into ancestry and permeating society at large. Education has told us that crime and vice are the work of criminals and vicious men; but science will prove that criminals and vicious men are the result of crime and vice.

Education has neglected the moral development of boys and young men. Educational methods and ideas should be the most progressive of all, yet the longest and narrowest and deepest ruts in history have been made by educators. For four centuries Education has been straining the memory, instead of training the mind and will; burdening the brain with antiquated data, instead of developing it into its highest possibilities.

The great teacher, Froebel, illustrated a moral as well as intellectual principle when he said: "All that does not grow out of one's inner being oppresses and defaces the individuality of man; instead of developing nature it makes it a caricature." Shall we never cease to stamp human nature, even in childhood, as we do coins, instead of aiding it to develop itself according to the natural laws of life?

Social influences lead multitudes of young men astray. The social faculty is perhaps the strongest power that actuates life. Society is the union of all opinions, motives, habits and desires, and its force is irresistible. The kings and princes of society rule the world. Wherever they go mankind is sure to follow. The social realm stands next to religion in importance. It is the duty of organized society to destroy the evil influences of the theatre, the ballroom, the club, the billiard and pool room, the saloon and the immoral resort. Future history must be chiefly social.

The general drift of fashionable life is toward a compromise of morals. That high reverence for chastity and virtue, which is the only safe standard, is being constantly assailed. There is no large city, and few large towns, where nightfall does not open clandestine resorts where boys and young men are made welcome and ruined. These places touch the social side of young men and capture them wholesale. A prominent educator says: "More boys and young men are ruined by questionable social retreats in our cities than by the saloons." The teacher of a class of young men in a city Sunday School, sometime since, discovered

176

that one of her scholars was visiting some low dens of iniquity. She decided to investigate the habits of her entire class and found that every one was doing the very same thing. Were the truth unearthed, many other teachers would be equally surprised. That such influences live and thrive and multiply and grow more alluring, more active and desperate, should not mark the progress of civilization. That the socially gifted do so little to counteract such influences by wholesome, elevating recreation, shows a serious flaw in our social system.

Legions of young men go wrong because it is so easy. They are ruined because the way is so short. It takes very little to wreck a life. "The worst man is seven-eighths exactly like the best man." A disease of one organ sickens the whole body, and a flaw at some vital point of the moral economy is ruin. The worst rascal, rogue, or reprobate is often the best and brightest man warped or weak at some vital spot. The difference between the criminal and the judge, the prisoner and the jailor, may be extremely slight. The dividing line is crossed by thousands unconsciously. Vices are too strong to be broken before they are great enough to be seen. "It is only three steps to ruin." The first step is subtle and short. It is simply a change of ideals, a slight deflection

of the vision, a revelry of the imagination, a
trivial turn of the footsteps. Drummond says:
"When we see a man fall from the top of a
five story building we know death is sure before he falls a foot." The same law applies
to the moral nature. When a young man allows his energies to cool, and he yawns and
drawlingly says, "Oh, well, life leads to nothing worth striving after," he has taken the first
step to ruin; he has lost his grip upon his
highest possibilities. Nine-tenths of the lost
were ruined just at this point.

When it is remembered that all evil influences work together in absolute harmony, that
in their union their strength is multiplied,
then, and then only, is their power appreciated.
The forbidden fruits of the modern Eden are of
endless variety. No taste, fancy or desire is
allowed to remain unsatisfied. Temptations
were never so abundant, never so subtle, never
so powerful as now, and perhaps young men ·
were never so poorly equipped to withstand
them. By inheritance, by birth, by education
and by experience the young men of America
are morally weak. They are, to a deplorable
degree, willing prey. While this is true there
was never such a determined and persistent
effort to ensnare them. More than ever before capital is invested, energy enlisted, and
business ability arrayed in schemes and enter-

Why Young Men Go Wrong.

prises to allure and ruin them. Young men have become a necessity—a staple commodity —in the markets of sin. Satan has a money interest in them. In the conflict between right and wrong for the character and souls of young men, wrong occupies the vantage-ground. To the interests of wrong they are a source of profit; to the cause of right, they are too often an expense. Wrong panders to their appetites and passions, while right demands their self-denial and forbearance; wrong is satisfied with indolence and extravagance, while right demands industry and economy; wrong is pleased with ignorance, while right insists upon knowledge; wrong gives what is wanted, right allows only what is needed; wrong can thrive upon weaknesses, while right depends upon strength; wrong accepts young men as they are, shows them the world and the glories thereof, and says: "All these things will I give thee," while right demands a clean heart and a new creature; wrong gives freedom and license, right enforces law and imposes duty; wrong is willing to deceive, cheat, beguile, mislead, lie, gull, tickle, please, promise everything, or grant anything, while right is honest, truthful and just; wrong is reached by a thousand paths, right is reached by only one.

While evils are legion and working in harmony day and night, seven days in the week,

the forces in the cause of right are confused
by divisions and frustrated through lack of
zeal and courage. Throughout the entire realm
of human influences are found causes, powerful
and persistent, which impel young men to ruin.
The pathways downward fairly bewilder with
music that enamors and with excitement that
enchants. Subtle enticements and seductive
charms, mantraps, soothing wiseacres, artful
wiles, wolves in sheep's clothing, blind and
perverse teachers, deceptive by-ways, false be-
liefs, perambulating, devouring demons, intimi-
dating and tyrannical powers flourish, fascinate
and hold dominion upon every side. While
the young men of America, thoughtless and
credulous, become willing victims of these be-
guiling influences, those who are fortunate
enough to escape too often stand aside and view
the havoc wrought with complaisant supine-
ness, too self-righteous to feel implicated and
too selfish and cowardly to lend a helping hand.

CHAPTER VI.

Paying the Piper.

Can one go upon hot coals, and his feet not be
burned?   *Solomon.*

> "He cannot plead, his throat is choked,
> Sin holds him in her might;
> And self-condemned, he slideth down
> To an eternal night."

"Those who dance must pay the piper."

I doubt whether the ferocity of the battlefield is as
merciless as is the remorseless onslaught of unscrupulous passion.   *Julia Ward Howe.*

Secret sins and kindred vices yearly ruin more con-
stitutions than hard work, severe study, hunger, cold,
privation and disease combined.
                              J. H. Kellogg, M. D.

Man is first startled by sin; then it becomes pleasing, then easy, then delightful, then frequent, then
habitual, then confirmed. Then man is impenitent,
then obstinate, then he is damned.—*Jeremy Taylor.*

Do we not all know what it is to be punished by
Nature for disobeying her? We have looked round
the wards of a hospital, a prison, or a madhouse, and
seen there Nature at work squaring her accounts with
sin.   *Henry Drummond.*

"What havoc hast thou made, foul monster, sin?

In the great majority of things, habit is a greater
plague than ever afflicted Egypt.   *John Foster.*

CHAPTER VI.

PAYING THE PIPER.

THE forces which have been shaping the history of our nation during recent years have made but little noise. The destroying elements in our midst have been wont to operate in seclusion and in silence. Waving harvest fields, laden with abundance, have made beautiful the face of our land, and the engrossing activities of manufacture and commerce are seen upon every side. We have been filled with the comforting thought that America is an invulnerable embodiment of peace, prosperity and power.

A nation, however, does not consist simply of an extensive wealth producing territory and a multiplying number of people. It is the intelligence, the industry, the character and the morals of individuals that decide the stability and insure the permanency of a nation.

The evil habits, vice, and immoralities which prevail to such an extent among young men cannot exist without a corresponding evil and

183

Manhood's Morning.

destructive influence upon the happiness and welfare of the people.

Only to the smallest degree is it possible to know how injurious and destructive to happiness, success and life are the evil habits to which so vast a multitude are addicted. People generally are imbued with the impression that at a certain age it is to be expected that young men will sow a crop of wild oats, and that in due season they will return to rectitude and no harm come from it. Men and women cry aloud against every other form of viciousness, except those sins which belong especially to young men. Regarding these a strange silence prevails. A peculiar and voluntary charity shields this unsavory realm of iniquity, and it is allowed to strut through the land blighting, killing and damning—a perpetual devastating carnage—and yet, aside from the curse of strong drink, we hear but little of the subject.

I feel fully certain that questions relative to intemperance, vice and immorality belong almost exclusively to young men. Justice demands that my position be made plain at this point. I have maintained that the period of young manhood is different from that which follows. In nothing is the difference so strongly marked as in the matter of habit. Men who have grown old in habit will not,

as a rule, ever change. There are, for illustra-
tion, thousands of excellent Christian men using tobacco. Its use with them has become almost organic. These men have my sympathy,
not my censure. Most of them deplore their
habit but it holds them in bondage. My father
was an inveterate tobacco user, but if he
caught either of his three boys using it, the rod
well applied, was the penalty. The fact that I
do not use it is to his credit; the fact that I
hate its use is a natural inheritance. Perhaps
it was not wrong for him to use it, but it
would be wicked for me to do so. There are
multitudes of men, noble Christian men, who
have grown old in the habit. They will never
abandon the habit, perhaps it never has and
never will become a matter of right and
wrong with them; but for young men to imitate them is entirely different. The light, the
science, the Christianity, and the needs of this
new age pronounce these things injurious and
wrong, and to become victims to them is sin.

We are told that "The wages of sin is death."
When death and the conditions which lead to it
are seen upon every side, searching for the
cause becomes a paramount duty. It is claimed, by competent observers, that the American
people are not living more than two-thirds
as long as they should. This means that on an
average more than fifteen years are cut off from

each human life. Man can no longer afford to
live in either ignorance or error. If advantages
lie hidden before him, it is a duty to grapple for
them; if pitfalls bestride his pathway, it is
wicked to blindly fall therein.

The time has come when timid, cowardly
language should cease, and when young men
should be told the truth regarding vice and destroying habits. Wherever there lives the soul
of a patriot, there should be found a fearless
champion of a cleaner, purer manhood. From
one border of our nation to the other an aggressive and relentless warfare should be waged
until a clearer and more wholesome moral atmosphere prevails among the young manhood
of the nation.

Irreverence, disrespect, vulgarity, obscenity,
the use of tobacco, intemperance, immorality,
personal defilement, licentiousness, gambling
and profligacy are in their very nature far-
reaching and destroying. All of these evils are
associated and work together, and thus united,
they form the gigantic and devastating curse
of the age. War, pestilence and famine combined sink into insignificance when compared
with the evil habits and wicked practices of
young men. They are direct and powerful
destroyers of the race, and wherever they prevail manhood becomes impaired in both body
and mind, and depraved in motive power and

will. Vice, like misery, seeks companionships, and when it gains a foothold in one form it never rests until every morbid appetite and evil desire have wrought their deadly work.

Profanity and vulgarity are twins. As a rule, they are the first-born among the vices. There may be men who are victims of these habits and yet maintain a high degree of moral integrity, but they are few. The influence of either is vile and dastardly. They are the first lessons taught in the devil's school, and to thousands they are the first steps on the road to perdition. They are Satan's gift cards and cost neither money, thought nor effort. To the victim they bring neither pleasure, satisfaction nor profit. Why men are profane and vulgar is as astounding as it is incomprehensible. That so many young men indulge in these habits only proves that they are so filled with the spirit of sacrifice that they are willing to work for the devil without pay sooner than be idle.

Nothing is more universally condemned than these two vices. They not only pollute the intellect, but the character and life. They rapidly become fixed habits, and are among the most difficult to overcome. They corrupt the imagination and more young men are ruined from evil imaginations than from passion. Napoleon said: "Imagination rules the world," and surely it moulds the individual character.

Manhood's Morning.

These habits breed coarseness and bad manners; they destroy the finer sensibilities; they turn chivalry into cowardice, and transform clean noble-hearted men into scandal-peddlers and virtue-pirates. Vulgarity is an unfailing sign of a depraved conscience, and profanity of a guilty one. Chaste and refined language never mix, and seldom alternate with debasing speech, and from such elevating thoughts stand aloof. These vices quickly rob young men of self-respect; God is driven from the heart, and the door opened for all manner of evils. Those so addicted cease to go to church, sneak out of the Sunday-school and sheepishly avoid every approach of refinement and virtue. Vulgarity is the passport to the brothel as profanity is to the saloon. Vulgarity leads young men by the legion into self-defilement and licentiousness, and profanity mocks and stifles their remorse. The vulgar and profane man is more than half ruined, and the remainder of the way is the devil's play-ground. Profanity and vulgarity form the hot-bed in which revel not only sensuous desires but wanton practices. They coil their slimy forms about the purity of womanhood and the virtue of manhood, and drag them into the pit of carnal indulgence, the end of which is disgrace and hell. A young man saturated with vulgarity and profanity breeds more contagion than if he had the small-pox.

Paying the Piper.

He will contamniate and infest an entire neighborhood in an incredibly short time. One such young man will do more damage than a dozen topers or a score of thieves. That these two vices have become fixed habits in our national life is one of the nation's most lamentable misfortunes.

The evil effects of tobacco are deep-seated and sure. Especially is this true when it is used by the young. The strength and usefulness of young men depend upon the full and perfect development of their physical, intellectual and moral natures. Nothing interferes with this more surely than the use of tobacco. Like all narcotics, its use has a deadening effect upon the moral sense, especially in young persons. Among all the evil habits to which Christian nations are addicted the use of tobacco in its direful effects surely takes a front rank. Liquor is the only agent that equals it and this might be seriously questioned. From much observation and careful study of the subject, my own opinion is that tobacco is one of the greatest enemies to the human race in the world, at the present time. The subtleness of its charm, the insidiousness of its action, the almost universal manner in which it is used and the deep-seated and lasting effects which surely follow its use, have no parallel regarding any other agent, in human history.

Manhood's Morning.

The use of tobacco clogs the intellect, shatters the nerves, lessens the ambition, saps the brain, interferes with bodily development and the mental vigor of all growing boys. It tends to create a thirst for strong drink, and its excessive use has been known to cause nervous dyspepsia, heart disease, sore throat, cancer of the mouth, throat and stomach, nasal catarrh, insanity and imbecility, and to sap the foundations of manliness and virtue. Nothing will so surely destroy the sense of honor and make liars and thieves of boys and young men as the use of tobacco. The record of a certain court shows that out of 700 convicts, 600 were there for crimes committed under the influence of liquor, and 500, of the 600, testified that the use of tobacco brought them to the drink habit. In France its use is prohibited in military schools. Observations made at Harvard, Yale and Princeton Colleges prove conclusively that no student who uses tobacco is ever at his best, physically or mentally.

I have never known but one physician of prominence to publicly recommend the use of tobacco, and he has spent two years of his life in an asylum on account of dissipation. Hon. Cornelius Walford, author of the *Insurance Cyclopædia,* one of the world's best authorities, says: "I believe tobacco to be a more insidious stimulant than alcoholic beverages. It can be

Paying the Piper.

indulged in more constantly without visible degradation; but surely it saps the powers of the mind. Until mankind can rise above beer and tobacco, the race will remain degraded as it now is, mentally, socially and physically." Says the eminent Dr. Willard Parker: "Tobacco is ruinous in our schools and colleges, dwarfing both mind and body. Tobacco is doing more harm in the world than rum. It is destroying the race." Prof. Spencer, of The Spencerian Business College, who has had under him over 50,000 scholars, says that the effects of tobacco are "premature age, shattered nerves, mental weakness, stunted growth and general physical and moral degeneracy." Says Prof. Mead, of Oberlin College: "The tobacco habit tends to deaden the sense of honor." Dr. Stowell, author of *Essentials of Health,* says: "Deceit seems to be a born companion of the boy and his cigarette. Boys who would not be guilty of telling a falsehood on other matters, soon find it easy to lie about this habit." At a meeting of the leading physicians of Philadelphia it was declared that "Cigarette smoking is one of the vilest and most destructive evils that ever befell the youth of any country; its direct tendency is to a deterioration of the race." Dr. W. Seaver, of Yale College, who has made careful and extended observations, says: "No young man can use tobacco without injuring

Manhood's Morning.

himself seriously." Dr. A. Arthur Reade, in
his Symposium, *Study and Stimulants*, says:
"It is truly remarkable that out of twenty men
of Science only two smoke, one of whom, Prof.
Huxley, did not commence until forty years of
age." Regarding its use by young men he
adds: "To them it is bad in any form. It poi-
sons their blood, it stunts their growth, weakens the mind and makes them lazy." The eminent author, J. D. Steele, Ph. D., says: "The
young man who uses tobacco deliberately di-
minishes the possible energy with which he
might commence the work of life." The testi-
mony of Prof. J. A. Kellogg is: "The results
of no vice are more certainly transmitted to posterity;" and that, "the children of such men
are robbed of their rightful patrimony and enter
upon life with a weakly vital organism, with a
system predisposed to disease and destined to
premature decay." The evidence of Thomas
Jefferson is: "The culture of tobacco is pro-
ductive of infinite wretchedness."

The American Indians, though in some respects favored, are, and for centuries have been,
a savage race. They are without self-respect,
ambition, or power to appreciate civilization.
They are cold-hearted, revengeful and possess-
ed of an uncontrollable appetite for whiskey.
As a cause for their peculiar and apparent
hopeless condition, tobacco stands almost alone.

Paying the Piper.

Indeed its use has been their one great vice.

Hundreds of women die every year, and thousands become nervous wrecks through sleeping with tobacco-saturated husbands. In no instance are the sins of the fathers more surely visited upon the children than in tobacco using. It produces in the offspring an enervated and unsound constitution which lessens the physical resistance and invites disease and death. It not only leads young men to the drink habit but holds them there. Signing the temperance pledge, in almost every case, proves a failure unless tobacco is included in the reform.

In thousands of cases where liquor is recorded, in newspapers and courts of justice, as the cause of crime, tobacco, and not alcohol, is really the guilty substance. In many cases it is doubly guilty—it leads to the drink habit and then makes the drunkard criminally desperate. My observation leads me to believe that the tobacco habit is more difficult to abandon than the liquor habit.

The fact that a few men use tobacco without apparent injury is no argument in its favor. Some men are invulnerable. They are not impressionable. They can go among small-pox or cholera; they can live amidst malaria or contagion with impunity. Their power of resistance is perfect; but such men are few. They

193

belong to the frugal, solid stock of the past, rather than to the active, nervous temperaments of the present generation.

The effects of Intemperance are constant and terrible. A conservative estimate of the annual number of deaths caused by intemperance in our nation is at least one hundred thousand. The majority of this vast army are young men. They represent the noblest, brightest, most lovable and promising of our manhood. It is nothing less than murder, wholesale, public and deliberate.

The use of alcoholic liquors causes a long list of diseases and morbid conditions which not only destroy life but cause untold misery among the people. Their use greatly lessens physical resistance. Those who drink stand surgical diseases badly. Such diseases as typhoid fever, pneumonia, consumption, rheumatism, dysentery and other debilitating maladies prove a scourge among the intemperate.

The use of alcoholic liquors directly causes apoplexy, paralysis, vertigo, both hardening and softening of the brain, delirium tremens, dementia, insanity, consumption, congestion of the lungs, fatty degeneration, nervous and valvular diseases of the heart, diseases of the blood, dyspepsia, catarrh and ulceration of the stomach and bowels, congestive sclerosis or hardening of the liver, diabetes and Bright's disease.

194

Paying the Piper.

Not only does it cause organic disease in every organ of the body, but it enormously increases the death rate among those who seem to escape visible evil results from its use. It not only kills openly and boldly, but gradually and secretly. The death rate among those exposed to the temptation to drink, while at their daily work, is more than twice as great as among those not so exposed. The death rate among temperate young men between the ages of fourteen and twenty-eight is not over six to ten per 1000, while among those addicted to drink it reaches from fifteen to thirty per 1000. Therefore, if one-half of the young men of America drink, it means that over 90,000 young men fall, every year, victims of the drink habit. The death rate among bar tenders is three times as great as among those engaged in agricultural pursuits. Those who have studied the subject claim that from eight to ten per cent. of the deaths occurring among men is due to the use of liquor.

It might be questioned, however, whether or not death is the worst result of intemperance. It is often, apparently, a greater curse to the living than to those whom it destroys. To none does it prove so great an evil as to young men. No drinking young man can attain to his best, either in body, mind or will. In becoming slaves to the habit young men forfeit self-respect and the confidence of others. No matter what may be a young man's attainments, abilities or ambition if his reputation must be labeled, "but he drinks," the chances are all arrayed against him. Those who are intemperate are tactitly branded, not by law, but by society, by opportunity and by business enterprise. Nothing so destroys the higher possibilities of young men. It forces them into lives of menial drudgery, disgrace and poverty. Nothing so thoroughly destroys their usefulness, or so quickly carries them beyond the realm of opportunity and possible success. The effects of alcohol upon the mind are ruinous. It perverts and weakens the memory, it sours the disposition, it arouses jealousy and suspicion and inflames the temper; it drives out the man and enthrones the brute and the beast. The young man who drinks becomes, in part, at least, a moral imbecile, and is never to be trusted. Such persons voluntarily ostracise themselves from elevating society and from desirable and ennobling avocations, and by being individually demoralized, they seek positions beneath where they would otherwise belong, and thus betray and embarrass the whole scope of enterprise and labor.

Personal and Social impurity is a formidable scourge. God intended that the bodies of young men should be clean, and that their lives should be pure, and there are no sins upon which He looks with more disfavor than upon personal defilement and licentiousness.

Secret sin is the greatest curse of blossoming manhood. It takes the glow from the cheek, the brightness from the eye and the life-blood from the veins. Nothing so destroys the will-power and vital energy. Under its influence the habits become slovenly, the appetites morbid and perverted, the muscles flabby and weak, the disposition insipid, the spirits melancholic and the whole demeanor sheepish, reclusive and embarrassed. It weakens the intellect and impairs the memory; the blood becomes thin and chilled and the countenance expressionless, betraying a guilty conscience and a depraved mind. It takes the native skill from the hand and the appreciation of the beautiful from the mind. Such young men lose personal magnetism and attractiveness, society ceases to appreciate them, and they avoid refined and elevating companionships. Thus isolated they become willing and helpless victims to every form of vice. The habit leads to insanity, melancholy, sterility and general decay. . It is thorough in its work, and finally destroys every faculty and every virtue which adorns and makes attractive, forceful and noble the estate of manhood. Says a famous writer: "Once the habit is formed, and the mind has positively suffered

from it, there would be almost as much hope
of the Ethiopian changing his skin, or the leop-
ard his spots, as the victim abandoning his
vice. The sooner he sinks to his degraded rest,
the better for himself and the world."

The evil effects of *licentiousness* are constant and sure. The devil palms off wanton indulgence as the very essence of worldly pleasure, and too many young men, allured by the
cruel deception, waste their substance following
strange women. They "go straightway as an
ox goeth to the slaughter" only to "mourn at
the last when their flesh and their bodies are
consumed."

When a young man gains a carnal knowledge
of a woman he surely ignites the flames of an
earthly hell. No matter whether it be gained
by deceiving some pure but trusting and affectionate girl, or by following the way of some
professional harlot, it will invariably prove an
indellible stain upon the nobler constituents
of character, and the memory of the deed will
forever gnaw the conscience. Carnality in-
jures a young man just as much as it does a
young woman. The fact that he is more likely
to escape public censure only tends to transform him into a more foolish brute, and into a
more villainous and cunning knave. When
such a man leads some pure sweet girl to the
marriage altar, the ghost of his sin will be

198

Paying the Piper.

there. When he drinks from the fountains of wedded bliss it will pollute, with bitter dregs, the sacred cup. When his children play and sing around his fireside, their innocent voices will meet a haunting and blighting echo within his soul.

By leading impure and dissolute lives, young men not only ruin their own health and shorten their own lives but threaten the degeneracy of the entire race. Until a higher standard of public morals prevails, it will not be safe to consider young men other than enemies to society and a constant menace to the American home. The effects of their sins are a scourge to the race which will inevitably grow more deep-seated and disastrous until the ravages are stayed by a social reform.

No diseases are so loathsome and incurable as those contracted through sexual transgressions. The man polluted by venereal disease is a walking contagion. His presence is a constant danger to health and life. There are, all the time, thousands of young men in our nation whose bodies are filled with consuming rottenness—vile, accursed and communicative —the result of sensuality. If they were cattle, instead of human beings, the health authorities, in behalf of public safety, would demand that they be killed and their polluted carcasses burned or buried beyond the reach of buzzards.

Manhood's Morning.

It would not be safe to tan their hides for shoe-leather. But such men court and marry pure, innocent girls, and raise families of children and give to them an enfeebled vitality and the germs of loathsome disease as an inheritance.

In some countries of the world the ravages of venereal diseases have risen to the magnitude of a plague. During a single year there were admitted to the hospitals of the United Kingdoms of Europe 21,965 cases of venereal disease, and in over 11,000 cases the malady showed itself in its very worst form. That it prevails in our own land, chiefly in large cities and manufacturing centres, every physician knows. It is found among all conditions of people and visits alike the hovel and the palace. Nothing is more terrible than the remorse which these diseases are sure to bring. Quacks reap a golden harvest from the victims—in their filth of body and ignominy of soul these terror-stricken wretches swarm around arrant fraud like moths about a lighted candle.

Upon nothing has God pronounced judgments more severe than upon licentiousness. The Bible is full of denunciations regarding it. "Be not deceived" says the Apostle: "neither fornicators nor adulterers shall inherit the kingdom of God." Says the wise man: "None that go unto her return again;" they shall "mourn at the last when their flesh and their

200

Paying the Piper.

body are consumed." The bold and practical Apostle said: "When lust hath conceived it bringeth forth sin, and sin, when it is finished, bringeth forth death." Well might the inscription, which Dante has inscribed over the gate of hell, be placed over the pathway of every young man who seeks for pleasure in sensuous indulgences:

"Through me you pass to the city of woe,
Through me you pass into eternal pain,
Through me, among the people lost for aye.
    *   *   *   *   *   *   *
All hope abandon ye who enter here."

Sexual indulgence is never necessary for health. While it is not claimed that this is a medical book, I wish to discuss this subject from a professional standpoint. Thousands of young men are led to believe that their manly vigor and inherent passions require an outlet, and that sexual indulgences are conducive to health. Physicians who have not studied the subject deeply can, perhaps, be found who would sanction such a theory. No impression is more false. A chaste and continent life favors, in every way, good health. More than this; it is promotive of the highest strength, beauty and personal magnetism.

In order to gain the opinion of the Medical Profession upon this subject, a large number of

Manhood's Morning.

eminent physicians have been interviewed by
a careful investigator. Their unanimous opinion is in favor of a continent life. A declaration has recently been signed by over fifty physicians, occupying prominent positions as medical men and as Professors in colleges, stating
"that chastity—a pure continent life, for both
sexes,—is consonant with the best conditions of
physical, mental and moral health." Among
the long list of signatures appear such names
as D. B. St. John Rosa, M. D., LL. D., President New York Academy of Medicine; George
F. Shrady, M. D., Consulting Chief, Hospitals
of Health Department, New York City, and
Editor *Medical Record;* Prof. John H. Billings,
M. D.; Prof. Ephraim Cutter, M. D.; Prof.
John A. Wyeth, M. D., New York Polyclinic;
Andrew H. Smith, M. D., New York Presbyterian Hospital; Prof. Henry Dwight Chapin,
M. D., of New York Post-Graduate Medical
School and Hospital; Prof. R. C. M. Page, M.
D., New York Polyclinic; Prof. David Web-
ster, M. D., New York Polyclinic and Dart-
mouth College, and Prof. Eugene H. Porter,
M. A., M. D., New York Homœpathic Col-
lege.

Says Prof. M. L. Holbrook, of New York
Medical College: "How it ever came about that
any one, especially a physician, who sees the
evil results of unchastity, should believe it nec-

Paying the Piper.

essary to health is a mystery to me." Henry
C. Houghton, M. D., of New York Ophthalmic
Hospital, says: "Certainly; it is a sad comment
on our American civilization that there is any
debate on this matter." J. Mount Bleyer, M.
D., says: "It is my belief that most of the sui-
cides are due to these excessive practices in
both sexes. It is the business of the physician
to step in as a reformer, and begin to educate,
and to open the eyes of mothers, fathers, daughters and sons regarding the effects of sexual
overstimulation." Prof. Lyman B. Sperry, M.
D., of Carlton College, in his admirable book,
Confidential Talks with Young Men, says:
"No condition of an unmarried man demands,
or even justifies, from a physiological, or any
other standpoint, that he consort sexually with
any woman, or that he resort to any measure,
natural or unnatural, for the gratification of
his sexual desires. Complete abstinence from
sexual indulgence is not only *safe* for an unmarried man, it is the *only* safe course for him."
In reply to an inquiry, the eight Professors of a
Medical University recently signed a declaration stating: "We know of no disease or any
weakness which can be said to be the result of
a perfectly pure, chaste life."

*The combined costs of evil habits and vice
are beyond calculation.* It has already been
stated that evil habits are seldom practiced

singly. A few young men may have only one bad habit—nothing more—but such cases are exceedingly rare. The great mass—the millions—of men serve pleasure for all there is in it. Young America seldom does things by halves. When young men seek after pleasure, as a rule, they taste every fruit, drink from every bowl and enter every doorway. They follow every indulgence, satiate every desire—and reap all the consequences. It is the unchecked and wholesale surrender to evil habits and wickedness that must be measured.

Man was made to live a pure, natural life and the laws which govern his existence are so inexorable that every transgression incurs a corresponding punishment. "Whatsoever a man soweth that shall he also reap." He who thinks or plans otherwise mocks God. If twelve million young men sin, twelve million young men, or their posterity, in manifold greater number, must suffer in consequence.

"Though the mills of God grind slowly, yet
    they grind exceeding small;
Though with patience He stands waiting,
    with exactness grinds He all."

Within the vitals of the young men of America exist the forces which will some day be transformed into the future generations of the land. Young men are already the fatherhood

Paying the Piper.

of posterity. The fact that the embryonic
and proximate elements of a majority of the
countless millions, yet unborn, float in the ven-
om of nicotine—in the poison of alcohol—in
blood made hot by passion—under imaginations
that revel in lust—imprisoned in a realm where
God is blasphemed—where love is unhallowed, where virtue is jeered and where fatherhood is ignored—this fact, in its momentous
importance, stands paramount, unrivaled and
first. It is within these mysterious and primitive confines that the issues of life germinate
and receive their bent and predilections. Here
it is that unnatural affection, disobedience,
hatred of that which is good, selfishness and
perverse tendencies are born. Here it is that
the promises of God are bartered away, the
natural birthrights blasted and life's destinies
mortgaged to the devil.

Young men are infinitely more responsible, as
fathers, before their children are born than
ever afterward. The difference between the
good and the bad, the upright and the vicious,
the physically sound and the diseased is largely
a question of birth and ancestry. The only
way to train up a child in the way it should
go is to begin years before it is born, and this
lesson young men must learn. "In the iniqui-
ties of their fathers shall they pine away," said
the great Lawgiver. "Visiting the iniquity of

the fathers upon the children," is a Divine law. A thoughtless, perverse fatherhood forms the basis of untold misery and death. Whole families are becoming syphilitic, scrofulous and consumptive and dying out of existence, the latter disease carrying off over 300,000 annually. Whole families are becoming intemperate, profligate and morally depraved. Whole families are becoming nervous, insane and imbecile.

Scrofula and consumption are chiefly the offspring of ancestral venereal disease. While consumption in its fully developed stages exhibits bacteriological features yet the chief incipient cause is an enervated nervous system—a neurosis—that is becoming widespread. The same might be said of nasal catarrh which is so prevalent in our nation. That the American people have grown more tense and nervous every physician knows. Nervous prostration, nervous debility, neurasthenia, nervous dyspepsia and other neurosis have become extremely prevalent, and seriously threaten the vigor and strength of our national physique. A well marked characteristic of the present age is that an increasing number of people live close to the margin of ill health. One-third of the children born have not vitality enough to survive to adult age. Over one-half million persons die annually who, under the best possible conditions, should continue to live; and the large number constantly sick and invalid are becoming a reproach to civilization and progress.

The riciprocal and radiating influences of these conditions are seen everywhere. As a prop for debility, and as a palliative for ultra-natural pain, the people flock to stimulants, narcotics and sedatives. Not only alcohol and tobacco, but opium, chloral and other drugs that enslave are widely used. The consumption of opium has rapidly increased in our nation. At the present time from one-quarter to one-half million persons are *habitues* of the drug. It is claimed by good authority that opium, in all its forms, destroys more lives annually than liquor. Its effects upon the moral sense is ruinous to the extreme. Of course, no one thing is the sole cause of this almost universal trend of our national life. Climate, social customs, intense business activities, fashion and many other things play their part, but the primal and basic cause is unquestionably "wild oats" as sown by young men.

It is a significant fact that where dissipation and vice prevail, healthy and robust men are not so longlived as the more frail and delicate. The best swimmer is most likely of all to be drowned, and the most powerful man is apt to outdo his strength. So it is that, unless re-

strained by moral principle, the man most lav-
ishly endowed with vigor is of all most apt to
fall into ruin, and the most brilliant and gifted
are the most tempted to resort to artificial stim-
ulation. Life insurance companies are rapidly
finding out that it is not a man's physical condition and general health at any specified time,
but his habits and morals that most surely decide the question of longevity.

Bad habits and vice cause sex deterioration.
Young men are incomparably less moral than
young women. The disparity between the
sexes morally is apparent to all. A chief reason
for this is plain. They inherit the predisposition from their fathers. Vice and evil habits
have become a matter of sex; they are largely
confined to the male side, and heredity is disposed to keep them there. Consumption, rheumatism and many other diseases, unlike some
traits of character, are much more apt to go,
as an inheritance, from father to son, or from
mother to daughter, than to wander across the
lines of distinction made by sex. Each succeeding generation of young men that yields
to profligacy makes this hereditary tendency
more organic and its results more disastrous.
Male children are more apt to die in childhood
than female, due no doubt, to a similar cause.
When the age of manhod is reached the death
rate rapidly rises, which is much less marked

Paying the Piper.

among women. Seven times as many men as women die suddenly. It is within the power of young men—the coming fathers—and none others, to lessen and destroy the hereditary tendencies to vice and evil habits. That they do so little, or nothing at all, is an amazing neglect of duty. Far more attention is paid to the improvement of the stock among horses and cattle, or even among chickens and dogs, than to that of immortal human beings.

Evil habits cause young men to avoid wholesome and elevating companionships. From the moment a boy takes his first lesson in any form of vice until he is lost in utter ruin, the whole tendency is to forsake that which is good and seek that which is evil. Nothing will cause boys and young men to quit the church and other religious influences, to avoid female society and seek questionable associations like conscious guilt. The vulgar and profane feel uncomfortable except among their own chums. Those who use tobacco or drink instinctively seek isolation from those who are free from such habits. The smoking car accompanying all trains, the men's cabin on all steamers and the loafing facilities around all barrooms are the natural product of bad habits.

By being thus divorced from elevating influences young men come to lose all interest in religion, ignore the Bible, descrate the Sabbath, avoid female society and abandon moral restraints. They deny themselves the advantages of the salt of the earth and of the light of the world. They rapidly become like those with whom they associate and they become organically wedded to a low standard of morals from which they have no desire to depart.

On account of evil habits young men forfeit their influence for good. Their force in combating evil, on this account, is almost wholly annulled. A man's moral courage and his influence over his fellows are usually measured by the weakest spot in his character. As a class young men engage in no warfare against the great evils of the day. Lawlessness, dens of iniquity, speak-easies and deviltry of any and every sort may boldly and fearlessly operate, and go on unrebuked, if none but young men witness the exploits. Bad habits so harden young men that they can stand and view, with stoic indifference, the most debasing episodes of shame or the most flagrant carnivals of sin. They become only too willing to flock around and patronize such things as do flies about a honey-baited trap. Satan never fears young men, and wastes no time defending himself against them. While moral heroes and women are waging a relentless warfare against intemperance and vice, young men, crippled by guilt, stand afar off, without the necessary armor,

Paying the Piper.

moral courage, or strength to enlist in the conflicts.

When the great revivals of religion take place, or when temperance workers gather in signers to the pledge, it is not unusual that in a short time the altars are forsaken and the pledges broken and the last end of such saved and rescued is worse than the first. It may be set down as an invariable rule that the chief cause of these lapses of will power is due to the fact that evil habits exist which are more powerful than the efforts put forth to abandon them.

Evil habits and vice prevent marriage and the perpetuity of the home. Says a famous writer: "America is on the verge of an age of unmarried women, because young men do not earn enough to support wives, and there is such a craze for dissipation among them that women had rather go in stores for almost nothing than risk their future in the bonds of marriage." Said a noted lecturer recently: "The reason there are so few marriages is because there are so many young men in jails and penitentiaries; tramping the country and loafing on street corners; spending their money in saloons and in questionable resorts of pleasure and wasting the flower of their manhood in dissipation and idleness." There are more males than females born, but the number of girls who would make faithful and desirable wives outnumber the "good catches" among young men many times over. The modern girl is not preparing to get married, as of yore, but is training herself in order that she may live independently by earning her own living. When a young man fails to marry and support a woman in dignity as wife and mother, as he should, he has no right to find fault if she become his rival in the higher industries and professions and forces him into menial avocations or idleness. That our nation, during times of peace and plenty and when the home life ought to reach its highest development, should produce a crop of over 3,000,000 confirmed bachelors and a corresponding number of unmarried women; that the birthrate should decrease, which has hitherto been an unfailing symptom, a pathognomonic forerunner of national decay; that young men and young women, instead of entering matrimony and establishing homes and rearing families, should become rivals and antagonists in professional life, in store and workshop, furnish a condition demanding most serious concern. Man's first duty to woman is to see that she shall not be obliged to go out into the world to earn her own livelihood. It is not woman's, but man's fault, that she does not marry. She is foregoing her God-intended mission, not from choice, but because vice, bad

Paying the Piper.

habits and improvidence among young men have made it justifiable and wise for her to do so.

Evil habits pervert business and corrupt wealth. The liquor bill of the nation is about $1,200,000,000; the tobacco habit costs $800,-000,000; marketable sensuality in an organized form, follows as third among the expensive vices. The cost of crime is rapidly increasing and the constant drain upon mind and muscle and legitimate business has become a tax of gigantic proportions. This perversion of business, in the aggregate amounts to at least $3,-000,000,000, annually. About one million young men reach their majority every year and if this vast sum, which is worse than squandered, were made to flow into their hands it would give to each one *three thousand dollars* as a start in life. This constant outlay is the source of untold misery and poverty. Every dollar so spent is that much out of pocket with absolutely no equivalent in return.

In these days, when political and moral questions are so intensely discussed, the extent and sources of evil habits and poverty, and their relation to each other, are closely studied. It is claimed on the one hand that from fifty-five to eighty per cent. of the poverty in the nation is due to intemperance and vice; while on the other hand it is claimed that from fifty to sev-

Manhood's Morning.

enty-five per cent. of the intemperance and
vice we see is due to poverty. Says Josiah
Strong in *The New Era*: "Doubtless much poverty is due to drunkenness, and again much
drunkenness is due to poverty." Beyond question bad habits and vice are the first and deeper
cause and also more blighting and destructive
in their results. In all genuine reform the first
step must be to change the habits and life of
the individual. This all can do, and it is the
only way to begin to abolish poverty.

"Those who study physical sciences," wrote
Charles Dickens, "and bring them to bear upon
the health of men, tell us that if noxious par-
ticles that rise from vitiated air were palpable
to the sight, we should see them lowering in a
dense black cloud above such haunts, and roll-
ing slowly on to corrupt the better portion of
the town. But if the moral pestilence that
rises with them, and in the eternal laws of out-
raged nature, is inseparable from them, could
be discernible too, how terrible the revelation!
Then should we see impiety, depravity, drunkenness, theft, murder, and a long train of nameless sins against the natural affections and re-
pulsions of mankind, overhanging the devoted
spots, and creeping on to blight the innocent
and spread contagion among the pure. Then
should we see how the same poisoned fountains
flow in to our hospitals and lazar-houses, in-

214

Paying the Piper.

undate the jails, and make the convict ships
swim deep, and roll across the seas, and overrun vast continents with crime. Then should
we stand appalled and know that where we
generate disease to strike our children down
and entail itself upon unborn generations, there
also we breed, by the same process, infancy that
knows no innocence, youth without modesty or
shame, maturity that is mature in nothing but
suffering and guilt, blasted age that is a scandal on the form we bear. Unnatural humanity!
When we shall 'gather grapes from thorns' or
'figs from thistles'; when fields of grain shall
spring up from the offal in the by-ways of our
wicked cities and roses bloom in the fat church
yards that they cherish; then may we look for
natural humanity and find it growing from
such seed."

"The tissue of the life to be,
   We weave with colors all our own;
And in the field of destiny,
We reap as we have sown."

Vice and evil habits assail every interest
and every possession. Life, health, intellect
and will; religion, society, patriotism and fra-
ternities; wealth, success and prosperity, alike,
go down to ruin under their destroying power.
But who can measure the havoc of evil habits
and vice? Social and personal impurity has

been the subtle and devouring octopus of human history. Through its power empires and kingdoms, glorying in their strength and magnificence and surpassing in their wealth and culture, have fallen to pieces and gone down into oblivion. It was on account of impurity and vice that God destroyed the human race by the flood; it was for the same reason that Sodom and Gomorrah were blotted out of existence. Impurity, especially among young men, caused the overthrow of magnificent and mighty Babylon, cultured and classic Athens and powerful and aggressive Rome. It has done more to dethrone governments and nations, obliterate happiness and destroy life than despotism, war and famine combined. It is God's worst enemy and Satan's best friend. It turns the beauty of youth into a passing delusion, the strength of mature manhood into a fruitless struggle and old age into a vain regret. It transforms health and vigor into decreptitude, and in place of the virgin bloom and innocent radiance of young manhood it gives the hectic blush and the pallid outlines of guilt. It robs the eye of its fascination and lustre and daubs its sockets with a dull and expressionless blear. It plunders man of respectful gallantry and protecting chivalry and veneers him with sneaking effrontery and impudent "brass" and "cheek."

Paying the Piper.

"I waive the quantum of the sin,
The hazard of concealing;
But oh, it burdens all within,
And petrifies the feeling."

Impurity destroys the natural affections and the nobler aspirations and fills the soul with hatred and remorse. It shuts out love and hope and heaven and leaves man in darkness and despair. "Be not deceived: God is not mocked; for whatsoever a man soweth, that shall he also reap." "When lust hath conceived, it bringeth forth sin, and sin, when it is finished, bringeth forth death."

CHAPTER VII.

What Young Men Must Be.

Show thyself a man.—*David.*

"Call up thy noble spirit,
Rouse all the generous energies of virtue,
And with the strength of heaven-endued man
Repel the hideous foe! Be great, be valiant!
O, if thou couldst, e'en shrouded as thou art
In all the sad infirmities of nature,
What a most noble creature wouldst thou be!"

"FIRST BE A MAN."—*Rousseau.*

"Manhood is above all riches, overtops all titles and character is greater than any career."
Orison Swett Marden.

Be sure, my son, remember that the best men always make themselves.—*Patrick Henry.*

Our greatest glory is not in never falling, but in rising every time we fall.—*Confucius.*

The truest test of civilization is not the census, nor the size of cities, nor the crops; no, but the kind of man the country turns out.—*Emerson.*

The secret of success in life is for a man *to be ready for his opportunity when it comes.—Disraeli.*

The truest wisdom is a resolute determination * * * I have only one counsel for you—*Be master.*
Napoleon.

As there is nothing in the world great but man, there is nothing truly great in man but character.
William M. Evarts.

The reverence of man's self is, next to religion, the chiefest bridle of all vices.—*Bacon.*

220

CHAPTER VII.

WHAT YOUNG MEN MUST BE.

IN the making of history the forces that operate are constantly radiating into new fields. Every new epoch in our progress has brought out and emphasized new and noble traits of character. Men have been called upon to meet one crisis and then another and new and special duties confront each succeeding generation. Ignorance, superstition, despotism and war have all in turn, had their struggles and conquests and the world, surviving them all, is looking, with exultant hopefulness, into the future.

Symmetry of development has been a constant characteristic of our nation's history. With increasing national resources have come a demand for higher ideals in the individual. The liberties, which we enjoy have developed virtue, industry, education, talent, inventive genius and indomitable push and enterprise. The founders of the nation had an unswerving faith in their children and children's children. They so planned the country's destinies that inasmuch as they were faithful over a few things their posterity should be rulers over many things. They staked the future of the republic upon manhood and not upon wealth and commerce. Little did they know of the extent of field and forest and less of the wealth of mine and mountain. Virtue, intelligence, industry and independence were the pillars upon which the nation was founded and upon these must it rest forever.

In this new era the principle *"Quality rather than Quantity"* is being applied to men. The time has come when *being* something is an essential preliminary to *doing* something. The duties and successes of life have called men to a higher plane of activity. That so many refuse to be led is the chief cause of the discord, unhappiness and failure so common.

A new and more perfect type of manhood—a new personnel—is called for. The real worth and intrinsic value of a man does not consist of the abundance of his wealth but of a richly endowed and well poised personality. The most useful citizen is he who rises highest as an individual. He is most loyal to his country who is truest to his own integrity. The greatest friend to liberty is he who governs himself. The noblest patriot is not the mightiest, but the purest man.

The battles of the future will be unlike those of the past. The enemies of our nation to-day are not skirmishing in the distance with musket and cannon, but they are in our midst. They are "bone of our bone and flesh of our flesh"; they have been born upon our soil and have grown up with us and form an organic part of our national life. The tactics of future warfare will not consist in trying to get within shooting distance of some foreign or alien enemy but in getting the enemy far enough separated from our own bosoms to give it a telling blow. Our foes are no longer telescopic but microscopic, not hideous and repulsive but subtle and winning. Right and wrong are no longer national differences, with oceans and well defined border lines between. Men do not go out to meet treason, oppression and wickedness in open conflict, upon the field of battle, and conquer with sword, rifle and cannon. Good and evil commingle, and live and work and play together. They sit in the same pew and are schooled under the same curriculum. Indeed, the good and evil of modern times wrestle in the same breast and wage a relentless warfare within the same vitals, mind and heart.

To simply multiply in numbers will never make America great as a nation. Wealth that is concentrated, power that is selfish and dogmatic will never insure our safety. America's security must ever depend upon the character of its citizens.

Manhood's Morning.

Our ability to successfully and profitably enjoy liberty, peace and prosperity is being put to a crucial test. Mankind is called upon to govern itself. "We live in an age," said Edward Everett, "and in a country where positive laws and institutions have, comparatively, but little direct force. But human nature remains the same. The passions are as wild, as ardent and as ungovernable in a republic as in a despotism." Herein lies our danger. Men are called upon not to be slaves but to be freemen, not to serve but to govern, not to bow to oppression but to stand erect in the clear sunlight of liberty.

This is man's normal sphere but it is the most difficult to fill. His highest and ultimate sphere is not to toil and drudge but to subdue and to exercise dominion. The present is a new era in the world's history; it represents a triumph of liberty; it is a crisis in the history of manhood. The new epoch is one of peace and

"Peace hath higher tests of manhood
Than battle ever knew."

There is a growing desire among all classes of people for a more contented and prosperous age. The past with its records of war, oppression and suffering is rapidly losing its prestige.

What Young Men Must Be.

Human experiences have, so far, been little else than wandering in a wilderness and there is a widespread and honest search for a grand highway which shall lead to a more prosperous and equitable era. The popular mind and heart are dissatisfied. Out of conflicting thoughts and energies is expected to come forth an ideal condition.

No matter how much froth and sentimentalism there may be upon the surface, man remains thoughtful, practical and serious. The noise and apparent friction, occasioned by the rapidity with which we move, may make a few skeptical and pessimistic, yet there continues an unswerving faith in the future. Hope was never so firm and anticipation never so confiding as they are to-day.

> "FORWARD! ye deluded nations,
>   Progress is the rule of all:
> Man was made for healthful effort;
>   Tyranny has crushed him long;
> He shall march from good to better,
>   And do battle with the wrong."

Young men must make the most and best of themselves. Nobility of character has ever been the bulwark of nations. History teaches nothing more plainly than that progress and prosperity, require a corresponding improvement in the type of manhood. The grave-

Manhood's Morning.

stones of almost every former republic warn
us that a high standard of moral rectitude as
well as of intelligence is indispensable.

While human history runs back nearly six
thousand years, men are alive to-day who have
witnessed one-half of the world's progress.
As the world moves forward men are required
to move upward and develop superior qualities
of mind and character. America is demanding
the energy, force and strength of the strongest
of men; an energy, force and strength which
only the young possess, and which the young
attain only through self-sacrifice and determined effort.

When the world was young it judged men
by what they said; as it grows older it esti-
mates them according to what they do. "What
a man does is the real test of what a man is;
and to talk of what great things one would ac-
complish if he had more talent, is to say how
strong a man would be if he had more
strength." The world is seeking for men with
the strength and force of quality. It is demanding a manhood that believes what it now
doubts, that constructs what it now neglects,
that cultivates and saves what it now wastes;
that lays upon the altars of duty and loyalty
what it now sacrifices at the shrine of base indulgences and selfish greed.

There is at the present time an overwhelming

What Young Men Must Be.

glut of incompetency and a famine of available, desirable men. Young men are begging no harder for work than high grade positions are begging for competent men to fill them. The entire realm of supply and demand is so exact and rigid that only goods of standard merit are sure of finding buyers in the markets of the world, and when men are wanted only those who meet a certain standard of excellence find desirable positions. Goods in the stores of merchants are literally plastered over with quality marks. Those labeled "XXX," "A, No. 1," "Extra-superfine," "Unadulterated," "Genuine," "I X L," "Guaranteed," "All Wool and Full Width," or "Fast Colors," find appreciative buyers, while those without anything to recommend them become shop-worn and must be sold at the bargain counter or at auction to the highest bidder. So it is with hundreds of thousands of young men. They swarm into the great centres of manufacture and commerce, representing an indefinite capacity and many of them a questionable quality, and while those who possess a special degree of grit and ability gain positions and success, the majority become a drug in the world's busy marts only to be shoved aside and doomed to idleness, servitude and poverty.

A mistake made by too many young men is to imagine that they can act out in their lives the part of useful and exemplary citizens without embodying corresponding traits of character within their own natures. As none but a strong arm can strike a powerful blow and only a keen, analytical mind can solve abstruse mental problems, so it is equally true that it requires the presence of a well-trained moral character to exert a strong moral force. "The fountain cannot rise higher than its source," and the deeds of man, his real success and his deserved fame and honor can never be higher or greater than is the source of all these—the character of the man himself.

The hearts of men, more than their heads or hands, shape history. "Out of the fullness of the heart the mouth speaketh," and the mind and energies work out the achievements of life.

Multitudes of young men make a failure of life, not because the chances of success do not exist, but because the elements of success are not within them. If there is nothing *in* a young man he may live under the most promising conditions of health, wealth and opportunities; he may have greatness thrust upon him, yet his life will prove a failure. Such a person will never attain success. But if the elements of success are *in* a young man he may be born in poverty and obscurity, so much the better; he may be haunted by infirmity and disappointment, but these will not dishearten; friends may

228

What Young Men Must Be.

forsake him and foes embitter his life, but he braves the storm; he may meet difficulties and embarrassments, but he is bound to succeed in spite of these things. Indeed, in the face of a capable, determined and courageous man obstacles and disappointments are only boulders upon which to climb, and the bitter experiences of adversity and opposition are simply incentives to greater diligence and nobler efforts.

Young men must be diligent and progressive in business. Diligence is more than simply industry. It means working with the might; throwing energy, heart and life into what we do. An ox or a mule may be industrious but they are never diligent. "Diligence is the mother of luck," and is always the price of genuine success.

Nothing so recommends a young man to the experienced business man like honest diligence. Nothing so quickly severs confidence as a slovenly lack of interest.

There is need of a revolution in the prevailing personal business methods of young men. With a few rare exceptions they use no system whatever in the management of their individual finances. The loose and careless manner in which they fritter away their small early earnings is simply ruinous. The foundations of almost every really successful career has been humbly laid by saving small fragments se-

229

Manhood's Morning.

cured through industry, patience and self-denial.

When young men squander their first earnings, be they ever so small, as a rule, it becomes a fixed habit and they live and die poor. If the first chances to save are wasted future opportunities are apt to pass unnoticed. When a young man is working for his board and two dollars per week he is just as surely a *business man* as the bank president or the merchant prince. It is his duty, at the end of each week, to be able to make out a trial balance sheet, and, if possible, declare a dividend and increase his bank account as a capitalist.

By early adopting systematic habits of business young men receive the advantages of a most wholesome discipline. Earning money by honest work not only develops the muscle, but practicing economy and laying by a portion for the future is an intellectual exercise eminently elevating to the moral nature.

Young men must be vigilant for the right. What young men need most is to become enamored of humanity. What the world needs most is the love and sympathy of strong and brave men. The world has many reforms to be wrought, many crusades to be manned and many conquests in behalf of truth and justice to be achieved, and young men alone possess the power and endurance to conquer.

What Young Men Must Be.

Young men, more than any other class, should be interested in the effort to correct the evils of intemperance, crime and lawlessness. Tens of thousands, many of them the very choicest of their number, go down to drunkards' graves every year. An appalling multitude waste their health and earnings in supporting the dram shops of the nation and millions of them pale their cheeks, dwarf their bodies and sap their intellects through the use of tobacco. These millions of young men are the trusted friends and bosom companions of millions of other young men. They are held together by all the affinities of brotherly good-will, luxurious spirits and personal magnetism. They are at each other's elbows, they grasp each other's hands and cheer each other's hearts.

Old men and women, philanthropists and benefactors may preach and sing and plead and sympathize to rid the world of evils but they will not prevail. These warfares belong to young men. They must not simply help but they must *do* the world's reforms.

When Lincoln, in 1861, called for volunteers, the men of the North, in amazing numbers, enlisted within forty-eight hours. These men represented the strength, bravery and patriotism of the nation and more than one-half of them were under twenty-three years of age. Men are called for to-day, not in one conflict

simply, but in many. The nation is being robbed of its possibilities by evils and selfish ambi-
tions upon every side. Never was there a more
positive demand for strong, brave, patriotic
young men.

"God give us men, a time like this demands
Great hearts, strong minds, true faith and ready hands.
*   *   *   *   *   *   *   *
For while the rabble with its thumb-worn creeds,
Its largest professions, and its little deeds
Mingle in selfish strife, lo! freedom weeps,
Wrong rules the land and waiting justice sleeps."

*Young men must be pure in word, thought
and life.* Men will never be pure in life until
they better appreciate their own bodies, and especially their sexual natures. The body is the
temple of God, and, next to the soul, the sexual
nature is its chief occupant. The sexual nature give grace and symmetry to the body, elas-
ticity to the step, warmth to the blood, strength
to the heart, force to the mind, firmness to the
will, beauty and radiance to the face and enthusiasm and courage to the whole life. It
gives to the behavior the grace and gallantry
of the gentleman, to the emotions the instincts
and affections of lover, husband and father, and
to the countenance the image of The Divine.

Untold injury has been wrought by stigmatizing the sexual nature. Every boy, when he

232

What Young Men Must Be.

blooms into manhood, should be taught that he enters an holy estate. The passions are not to be despised nor blasted by sin, but held and appreciated as a sacred possession and as the most attractive, noble and magnetic expression of manhood.

Grant Allen, in "The New Hedonism" has beautifully and graphically described the sexual instinct: "Its alliance is with whatever is purest and most beautiful in us. To it we owe our love of bright colors, graceful forms, melodious sounds, rhythmical motion. To it we owe the evolution of music, of poetry, of romance, of *belles lettres;* the evolution of painting, of sculpture, of decorative art, of dramatic entertainment. To it we owe the entire existence of our esthetic sense, which is, as a last resort, only a secondary sexual attribute. From it springs the love of beauty; around it all beautiful arts circle as their centre. Its subtle aroma pervades all literature, and to it we owe the paternal, maternal and marital relations; the growth of the affections, the love of little pattering feet and baby laughter; the home, with all the dear associations that cluster around it; in one word, the heart and all that is best in it.

"If we look around among the inferior animals, we shall see that the germs of everything which is best in humanity took their rise with them in the sexual instinct. The song of the

233

nightingale or of Shelley's skylark is a song that has been acquired by the bird himself to charm the ears of his attentive partner. The chirp of the cricket, the cheerful note of the grasshopper, the twittering of the sparrow, the pleasant caw of the rookery—all these, Darwin showed, are direct products of sexual selection. Every pleasant sound that greets our ears from hedge or copse in a summer walk has the self-same origin. If we take away from the country the music conferred upon it by the sense of sex we shall have taken way every charm it possesses, save the murmur of the brooks, and the whispering of the breeze through the leaves at evening. No thrush, no linnet, no blackbird, would be left ; no rattle of the night-jar over the twilight folds, no chirp of insect, no clatter of the tree-frog, no cry of the cuckoo from leafy covert. The whippoorwill and the bobolink would be mute as the serpent. Every beautiful voice in wild nature, from the mocking-bird to the cicala, is the essence of the love-call; and without such love-calls the music of the fields would be mute and the forest silent.

"Not otherwise is it with the beauty which appeals to the eye. Every lovely object in organic nature owes its loveliness direct to sexual selection. The whole esthetic sense in animals had that for its origin. Every spot on the feathery wings of butterflies was thus pro-

duced; every eye on the gorgeous glancing
plume of the peacock. The bronze and golden
hue of beetles, the flashing blue of the dragon-
fly, the brilliant colors of tropical moths, the
lamp of the glow-worm, the gleaming light of
the firefly, spring from the same source. The
infinite variety of crest and gorget among the
iridescent humming-birds; the glow of the tro-
gon, the barbets among the palm blossoms;
the exquisite plumage of the birds of paradise;
the bulb-and-socket ornament of the argus
pheasant; the infinite hue of parrot and macaw;
the strange bill of the gaudy toucon and the
crimson wattle of the turkey still tell one story.
The sun birds deck themselves for their court-
ship in ruby and topaz, in chrysoprase and
sapphire. Even the antlers of deer, the twisted
horns of antelopes, and the graceful forms and
dappled coats of so many other mammals have
been developed in like manner by sexual selection. The very fish in the sea show similar
results of esthetic preferences. The butterfly
fins of the gurnard and the courting colors of
the stickleback have but one explanation. I
need not elaborate this point. Darwin has already made it familiar to most of us. Throughout the animal world almost every beautiful
hue, almost every decorative adjunct is trace-
able to the action of the sexual instinct. Animals are pleasing to the eye just in proportion

to the amount of esthetic selection that their mates have exercised upon them; and they are most pleasing of all when most sexually vigorous, especially at the culminating point of the pairing season. Tennyson's familiar lines give a new meaning when we read them thus, as illustrating the persistent thread of connection between the esthetic sense in man and animals:

" 'In the spring a fuller crimson comes upon the
        robin's breast;
In the spring the wanton lapwing gets himself another
        crest.
In the spring a livelier iris changes on the burnished
        dove;
In the spring a young man's fancy lightly turns to
        thoughts of love.'

"Oddly enough, the same thing is true in all probability in the world of plants. Flowers are either the sexual organs themselves, as in the golden acacia, the meadow rue and the willow catkins; or else they are the expanded and colored surfaces in the neighborhood of the sexual organs, intended to allure the fertilizing insects, as in the rose, the lily, the buttercup and the orchid. True, these expanded surfaces are not, like the tail feathers of the lyre-bird or the plumage of the kingfisher, the result of deliberate selection on the part of the species itself which displays them. They are product of esthetic preferences exerted by the bee or butterfly or brush-tongued lory. External organisms—birds and insects—have begotten them. Still, I hold that to any one who takes a wide and deep view of nature the fact itself is significant. In plants, as in animals, beautiful adjuncts tend to develop themselves in immediate relation to the sexual function, and hardly at all elsewhere.

"It is the same with fruits. Such exquisite objects as the pomegranate, bursting red through the rind on the tree; the orange, aglow among its glossy green foliage; the cherry, the plum, the mango and the currant; the purple bloom on the grape, the blushing cheek of the peach—what are they but the mature state of the ovary of the female flower?

"Look at nature as a whole, and we shall see how truly all this is so. The song of birds, the chirp of insects, feather and fur, crest and antlers, the may in the hedgerow, the heather on the hill side, the berries on the holly, the crimson fruit of the yew, the apple tree laden with the blushing blossoms in spring and with the blushing fruit in autumn, the great tropical flowering trunks in the forest, and the garrulous birds and bright insects that flit, flashing through them—all alike owe their beauty to sexual needs and esthetic preferences. If one goes on a country walk, almost every fair object that attracts the eyes, from the gorse to the lady-bird, from the stately heron to the daisy on the common, attracts them in virtue of some sexual adornment.

"I have pointed out already in my little book on the color sense that the most brilliant and decorative birds, insects or mammals, are, every one of them, either flower hunters or fruit eaters; and that thus the entire beauty of the organic world, with the sole exception of the death-tints of autumn, is wholly due to a sexual origin.

"Still less need I dwell on the share which sex has borne in the development of the sympathies and the domestic affections. The parent bird with the nestlings, the males which feed their sitting mates, the ewe with her lamb, strike the key-note of something higher than even the esthetic sentiment. Tenderness and pathos come in with the paternal and marital relation. The love of mate, the love of young have this origin. Think of the widowed wren that laments her lost partner; think of the love-bird that cannot consent to live when deprived of its companion; think of the very monkeys that refuse all food and die broken-hearted when the bodies of their dead mates are taken from them.

"Thus, even below the human level, we see that the instinct of sex has been instrumental

What Young Men Must Be.

in developing all the finest feelings which the lower creation shares with us or foreshadows parental responsibility for us. The sense of beauty, the sense of duty, paternal and maternal love, domestic affection, song, dance and decoration; the entire higher life in its primitive manifestation; pathos and fidelity; in a word, the soul, the soul itself in embryo—all rise from the love of the sexes.

"Human life shows us the same thing in a more advanced development. The tenderest and most pathetic element in life is love; round it all art, all romance, all poetry circle. The loveliest object on earth for the sane and healthy mind is a beautiful girl, a beautiful woman. The loveliest object art can represent in painting or sculpture is the nude male or female figure. Pure or half draped, it supplies the base of all ideal artistic representation. Man is beautiful; woman is beautiful; both are most beautiful in the budding period and plentitude of their reproductive power. And love, which in itself is the most sacred and beautiful thing in the world, linked on every side with the tenderest affection for father, mother, sister, husband and wife for son or daughter— . love thus lovely in its essence has begotten among all higher arts and all higher emotions."

There is a widespread impression that a pure and chaste mind is necessarily insipid, morose

Manhood's Morning.

and incapable of joy and pleasure. Just the
opposite is true. The sweetest and most precious joys are as delicate as the life and fra-
grance of the lily. God clothes the highest de-
lights and most enrapturing pleasures in spot-
less garments and he who besmirches them with
filthy tongue or lustful eye robs life's most sacred fountains of their sweetness and beauty.

"Self-reverence, self-knowledge, self-control,
These three alone lead life to sovereign power."

It is not only possible, but it is imperatively
necessary that the lives of men be as pure as
those of women. It is shameful and wicked
cowardice for men to erect a high standard of
virtue for their sisters and a low standard for
themselves. A pure life is the strength of man
as it is the beauty of woman.

"My strength is as the strength of ten
Because my heart is pure."

Purity of life is the palladium of earthly
happiness; it is the stronghold of religion and
the chief cornerstone of society. "He that
hath it," says Milton, "is clad in an armor of
steel;" and Shakespeare says, "It is the jewel
of my house, bequeathed down from my ancestors." It is "the mother of wisdom and de-
liberation;" "the window in the soul through

240

which young manhood hears the angels of heaven singing songs of peace and welcome over the birth place of its children."

Reverence of the sexual nature has done more for the world than either power or wealth. It is the divine finishing touch in making a gentleman and is the harbinger of all the graces, be they physical, moral or spiritual. It surounds its possesor by an earthly paradise, it make women appear angelic and lays upon the marriage altar a feast of love. God loves a pure man, and it is seldom such are found who are not genuine Christians. The lives of such men are a beatitude, blessing the generation in which they live and giving to the fibre of the race pure blood, invincible nerve and sterling qualities of mind and character.

Young men must be woman's loyal friend. Man and woman were created equal and neither was given dominion over the other. Every true man holds sacred the estate of womanhood. Genuine gallantry enthrones all women.

Young men are peculiarly interested in woman's welfare. The girls of America are their sisters; they will become their sweethearts and life companions and will some day be the mothers of the nation. Woman ministers at the very fountain of life and happiness. Upon her health, her intelligence, her piety, her patience and constancy, her temper and her beauty depend the comfort and success of mankind.

"Of earthly goods, the best is a good wife;
A bad, the bitterest curse of human life."

Of a good wife Jeremy Taylor says: "Her voice is sweet music, her smiles his brightest day, her kiss the guardian of his innocence, her arms the pale of his safety, the balm of his life; her industry his surest wealth, her economy his safest steward, her lips his faithful counselors, her bosom the softest pillow of his cares, and her prayers the ablest advocate of Heaven's blessings on his head." To merit such a gift demands that man's heart be pure, that his lips be clean and that his life be free from guile.

Young men must be religious. Of all the subjects which young men are called upon to consider religion is of first importance. Religion equally concerns the entire human race. I do not feel called upon to champion the claims of religion nor to write a single word to prove its existence. He who cannot read it in the lives and characters of men and women is willfully blind. The foe in America to-day is not open infidelity but neglect and indifference toward the subject of religion.

Religion is all it claims to be. It is not a

What Young Men Must Be.

sentiment to feed the emotional nature. It is a moral and spiritual force and supplies man's highest needs. Through it man learns the way of eternal life, through it he learns of virtue and faith, hope and love. It moulds the character and sweetens the life, it exalts all that is noble and establishes the brotherhood of man.

There are three cardinal things connected with religion about which it is the duty of every young man to exercise convictions. These three things are:—The Bible, The Church and The Sabbath Day.

The *Bible* is a young man's book. It is chiefly about young men—a record of their thoughts, their words and their deeds—and many of its teachings apply to them only. No book so upholds the supremacy of youth and young manhood. Threads of manly strength and vigor run through its pages from Eden to Patmos. It is written "to young men because they are strong." It is the only safe guide; the only perfect rule of life. "Wherewithal shall a young man cleanse his way; by taking heed thereto according to thy word."

The Bible refers to young men and youths over two hundred times. Its most striking characters are young men—young kings, young prophets, young apostles and young heroes. The prototypes of Christ were young men and Jesus Himself was a young man.

243

Manhood's Morning.

"From my youth up," was the certificate of character in Bible times. The whole realm of religious thought and activity needs resetting in a more youthful and magnetic life.

The Bible is not only a young man's book but it is our official standard. As long as America remains a Christian nation the Bible must continue as the light of its people. To ignore it is heathenism in the darkness of which virtue and liberty would not long survive.

The *Church* is essential to every young man. He who faithfully and regularly goes to church receives benefits incalculable. The pulpit, as a rule, is supplied with earnest, well educated Christian men and the Church furnishes an education of the highest order and much of it is specially adapted to young men.

The Church has a mission peculiarly its own. It is divine in its nature and perfect in purpose and plan. Other organizations teach and practice noble principles but they lack vital essentials and fail to meet man's highest needs. There is no substitute for the Church.

That the Church falls below what it should be none can deny. It lacks zeal, activity and spiritual power. That it lacks these things is the fault of young men. Except in rare cases it is not the fault of the ministry, the aged or the women. Too many young men are derelict, disloyal and lazy. The Church is being

244

assailed on account of their shortcomings. The weakest point, the greatest breach in the church to-day is the void made by young men. The Church is as essential in the nation as the political government, and it is as much the duty of young men to reverence it and labor in its behalf as it is to enlist in the cause of the nation in its time of peril.

The Church teaches not only spiritual truths, but patriotism, morality, ethics, refinement and culture. It affords the only desirable level where all classes and conditions meet as equals. It brings together the aged and the young, the learned and the ignorant, the rich and the poor and it is the greatest and most elevating social factor in the world. It creates the noblest incentives, it promotes the deepest friendships and affords to young men and women the safest and most desirable ground on which to meet, enjoy each other's company, fall in love and marry under the skies.

The *Sabbath Day* was made for man. Man needs it. The rest of one day in seven is just as essential to man's highest development as bread or sunlight or sleep. Man can do more work and better work by resting one day in seven than by continuous, unremitting plod. Without the rest of the Sabbath labor becomes degrading to morals and debilitating to body.

It would be a wise movement to make of

Manhood's Morning.

Saturday a universal holiday free from all general business and public service. All business that brings men in contact with each other and all manufacturing and general labor could easily be transacted in five days. This would give one day for domestic improvement, ornamentation, repairing and arranging the affairs of home, and one day for rest. It would give one much needed off-day and an opportunity to enjoy, without encroachment, one Sabbath each week. Domestic and home affairs would thus receive a much needed attention, and the Sabbath Day would be relieved of much of that intense business pressure which now squeezes the life almost out of it.

The Sabbath must not only be remembered, but it must be "kept holy." The influences of the Sabbath as a Holy Day are incalculably beneficial. It thus forms an oasis along the pathway of life. It inspires elevating and serious meditation. "The Sabbath Day," says Emerson, "is the core of civilization." Sabbath Days, when remembered and kept holy, are like the waves of the ocean which follow each other in graceful outline, lifting man above the level of ordinary life and carrying him nearer a higher and happier existence; but when forgotten or spent in desecration they are like the tempestuous billows which bewilder with their madness and hurry us on to destruction.

246

What Young Men Must Be.

The Sabbath Day is one of the corner-stones of the Republic, a charter legacy coming to us as a part of the organic life of the nation. Modern ideas and customs are however transforming it into a day of worldly amusement and dissipation. It is the duty of young men to arrest this tendency. From their ranks come most of the Sabbath breakers and it is their duty to maintain its sacredness. It should be used to promote natural affections and domestic fellowships; as a time for reflection and rest and as a day to promote morality, charity, piety and Christian worship.

To make clear the cardinal principles which underlie success in life, I have epitomized them into seven paragraphs, in the form of a pledge. I have endeavored to embody nothing that could well be left out, and left nothing out the absence of which would weaken a popular vow. It is adapted especially to young men between the ages of fourteen and twenty-eight.

This pledge has been submitted to a large number of competent men in various sections of the nation and it has been pronounced eminently opportune and practical.

Manhood's Morning.

YOUNG MAN'S PLEDGE.

(1) *I do hereby promise to faithfully and industriously endeavor to earn an honest living, to practice charity and liberality, and if possible save a portion of my income.*

(2) *I will lead a temperate life, and abstain from the use of tobacco in every form and from all alcoholic liquors as a beverage.*

(3) *I will not use vulgar or profane language, nor indulge in low or indecent conversation.*

(4) *I will strive to lead a pure life and in no way defile my body.*

(5) *I will at all times reverence womanhood and treat every woman with that respect due a sister or mother.*

(6) *I will keep the Sabbath day holy by avoiding all desecration and unnecessary labor, and I do promise to make the attendance upon the services of some church a habit of my life.*

(7) *I do promise to keep a copy of The Bible and familiarize myself with its contents.*

A pledge is simply an expressed plan of action to guide and direct the habits and efforts of life. Throughout all history, vows, promises and pledges have formed the basis of the noblest efforts and highest achievements. Few things have done more for man than pledge signing. It brings the otherwise impossible within the range of the possible and makes difficult things easy. It is an act which God recognizes and they are scattered all through the Bible history. Indeed, the Bible might be well considered as God's pledge to men. The life of Wendell Phillips was a pledge and he said, "Tens of thousands attest the value of the pledge. It never degraded; it only lifted them to a higher plane." "What we need," says the eminent Dr. Peloubet, "is a pledge signing revival." Over a million members of the Young People's Societies have signed a pledge during the past few years, and it has been to thousands of them not only a restraining but an inspiring and saving force.

The pledge here presented is reasonable; it is not meddlesome in politics or religion. It forbids no real pleasure or joy. It will be easy to keep. It is easier to break off all bad habits than simply one. The failure of the temperance pledge so noticeable is due to the fact that too many habits remain untouched. It is easier to quit both tobacco and liquor than either alone.

A pledge that is comprehensive, and which complements what is sacred and vital in manhood, secures the confidence and respect of

Manhood's Morning.

those who sign it, and it becomes, of itself, a
source of courage and strength. At best it is
humiliating to sign a pledge to be correct in
some particular spot, but to promise to be
clean, pure, square and upright, from head to
foot, is a matter of which to be proud. A
pledge embracing one idea tends to weaken
from the time it is made, but a vow to change
the whole life grows stronger and is finally invulnerable. Never were definite purposes and
fixed determinations regarding habits of life,
traits of character and plans of action more
needed among young men than now.

The signing and keeping of this pledge
would bring benefits incalculable to young
men. It would promote self-respect and the
confidence of others. Confidence, genuine and
whole souled, in boys and young men is the
"fatted calf" of civilization. Too many young
men are as beggars at the door of popular opinion. To gain the confidence of the public is the
first step to success. When young men secure
the full confidence of their superiors in years,
wealth and influence a bright day of prosperity
and rejoicing will be at hand.

The social effects of a pure and consistent
manhood are beyond measure. The most powerful disinfectant in the world is a pure young
man. When young men become chaste and
pure they will swarm forth, millions of them,

250

and inaugurate a new social era. Refined æsthetic tastes will develop and more wholesome and elevating forms of amusements will be demanded. A new market will be opened for the products of artistic and cultivated handicraft. A new prosperity, busy in supplying improved desires with improved supplies, will mark the steps of progress.

Keeping such a pledge would reduce the amount of sickness to a minimum. The death rate among pure, temperate, worthily occupied men between fourteen and forty is extremely small. Sickness, to such, during these years, unless inherited or of the contagious sort, is extremely rare. By leading pure and temperate lives, the physical resistance against disease, which is now so low among the intemperate and licentious, will become strong, minor ailments will disappear and the more serious and fatal diseases will respond much more readily to medical treatment. The delusion that it is the hand of Providence, instead of vice and wickedness, that strikes men down will be exploded.

Men will become firmer in muscle, stronger in bone, richer in blood, brighter in eye, sweeter in temper, keener in intellect, more courageous in will and more manly and spiritual in heart. They will become more magnetic, their personality will be more richly

251

endowed and gallantry will become a delight
and chivalry a second nature.

> "The reason firm, the temperate will,
> Endurance, foresight, strength and skill."

As men improve in habits hereditary influences become recuperative and constructive
and each succeeding generation find it easier
to do right. That ideal—the genius of law—
which makes it difficult to do wrong and easy
to do right will become the natural heritage
of citizenship. Good health and good manners might be made contagious. It is possible for young men to so purify and enrich the
elements of kinship that each succeeding generation will not only be stronger and wiser,
but will inherit a momentum, constantly increasing in force, towards physical, intellectual,
moral and spiritual perfection.

By adopting such principles as are set forth
in this pledge young men will meet the demands of the hour and become prepared to
lead in every department of thought and action. Pauperism, drunkenness, crime and
misery will disappear. Men will become better educated and more refined, they will wear
better clothes, use better language, seek new
joys and cultivate higher attainments. They
will grow more polite and sociable, more kind-

What Young Men Must Be.

hearted and charitable. They will become more independent and wealth will become diffused among the masses. Men will love with a holier affection and enjoy a happier and more contented career. This pledge aims in the direction of man's best hopes, noblest aspirations and highest and most useful possibilities, and if universally signed and consistently lived by young men, the effect would be to elevate them to their normal, legitimate and God-intended sphere, and to hasten the glad day when the kingdoms of this world shall become the kingdoms of our Lord and his Christ.

CHAPTER VIII.

What Young Men Must Do.

Be fruitful, and multiply, and replenish the earth, and subdue it.   *God.*

"Because thou art
    The struggler; and from thy youth
Thy humble and patient life
Hath been a strife
    And battle for the truth;
    Nor hast thou paused nor halted,
Nor ever in thy pride
Turned from the poor aside,
But with deed and word and pen
Hast served thy fellow men;
    Therefore art thou exalted!"

Where should any being find its highest blessedness but in the legitimate exercise of its highest power.
                                        Mark Hopkins.

It is no man's business whether he has genius or not; work he must.   *John Ruskin.*

The powers of man have not been exhausted. Nothing has been done by him that cannot be better done.
                                        Emerson.

God never sent any man on a fool's errand.
                                        T. DeWitt Talmage.

Ah! the key of our life, that passes all words, opens all locks, is not *I will*, but *I must*—I MUST—I MUST and I do it.   *A. H. Clough.*

If our civilization stands, this will not be because it is incapable of destruction, but because its sons and daughters, roused by its dangers, rally to its defense.
                                        Samuel Lane Loomis.

"Why, now I see there's mettle in thee, and even from this instant, do build on thee a better opinion than ever before."

256

CHAPTER VIII.

WHAT YOUNG MEN MUST DO.

EVERY young man in America was made for a purpose and that purpose was to do something. Not one lives who has not a mission, a duty to perform. Whether his talents be one or five, conspicuous or obscure, strong or weak, they were given him, not to bury, but to exercise and improve.

Young men must act for themselves. Each generation of young men are the pioneers of a new age. It always has been and always will be so. The rest of the world keeps step with its young men. When they march forward the world moves on; when they aim high and strive upward civilization advances; when they are loyally enlisted in the cause of right happiness and safety are assured to the people.

What is true of the world at large is distinctively true of America, and it was never so true of America as it is to-day. Emerson said: "As goes America so goes the world;" and another has added, with no less truth but with still greater force: "As go the young men of America so goes America." If these statements are true prophetic wisdom the future history of the world and the destinies of the human race are within the grasp of the young men of America. I accept the proposition as a sacred verity, and believe that the uppermost need of the hour is that young men awake to the duties and responsibilities which these facts impose.

It is useless for young men to sit down and grumble and lament over our business, financial and industrial systems, or our social, political or religious conditions. The wrongs and evils and unjust conditions that exist, and which have become a part of our national life, will never be argued nor resolved out of existence. The only remedy for these conditions is for young men to enter the various fields of action determined that better conditions shall prevail, and that the world shall receive the benefit of their strength, vigor and enthusiasm.

It is useless for young men to expect help from the rich and influential. It is worse than useless for them to wait for anybody's shoes. They need not hope to supplant or frustrate their superiors. They must plan and build their own fortunes and do it by reaching farther, climbing higher, digging deeper and striv-

What Young Men Must Do.

ing more unselfishly and constantly than those who are ahead of them.

Too much is being done already for many young men. Help is the last thing they need. Nothing spoils them so quickly. Thousands have been ruined by learning to depend upon others instead of themselves. The world should be laid upon their shoulders. The duties and perplexities of the world—its sufferings and its wrongs, its hatreds and oppressions, its ignorance and filth, its fossilisms and its perversions—should be heaped upon and piled around young men and they should not find pure air, comfort, rest, peace nor even sleep or bread until they earn it by digging and fighting their way out and trampling these things under their feet.

Young men must not stand upon the brink of life's business channels and shrink and shiver into despair, but they must plunge in, and through their own industry, grit and brains overcome all obstacles and win success.

Too many stand and beg for the crumbs that fall from the tables of the rich, and starve as they deserve. Young men are in duty bound to aim high and not be too easily pleased. Too many lives are wasted in hewing wood and drawing water and doing things out of date. Thousands seek work for their uneducated muscle while the world is looking for brains. They hunt in the dark and dingy corners of enterprise for jobs at starvation wages while the world is offering comfortable salaries and honor to men of worth and sagacity.

That so many young men find it difficult to secure employment is not always a cruel fate. Their ill success is often only a whip to spur them on to something better. When they get behind and separated from where they belong they must expect to suffer. When young men are thrown out upon their own resources it is simply the American Eagle stirring her nest and forcing "Young America" to shift for himself, to manage his own affairs and live independent of others.

Seeking employment in factories, stores and offices needs to be discouraged. Too many spend their lives in routine, automatic service, like so many machines. Such avocations lack permanency and tend to sap the higher qualities of mind and character. They rob men of the art and ambition required to venture into the more independent realms of action. By so doing they grow narrow and timid and distrustful of themselves, and stripped of their native pluck and ambition they sink their individuality and ability in the industrial monopolies of the nation. Every man should have a genuine and direct interest in his life's work—in its profits, in its management and in its gen-

What Young Men Must Do.

eral success. The hands of men should not only be employed but their brains and their hearts—their might—should have a living interest in what they do.

Young men must work. Persistent, concentrated work is the price of genuine success. Achievement is too often looked upon as the result of genius or luck. Genius is greatly overestimated and luck comes to but few. Ninety-nine young men in every hundred must depend for success upon their own energies. "A genius for hard work is the best kind of genius."

It is the general impression that orators, poets, inventors and others do not have to apply themselves. This belief has done much harm. It is claimed that Demosthenes, the world's greatest orator, had no talent whatever, but owed his success entirely to hard work. He was sickly born, nicknamed on account of ugliness, and stammered. He shaved the hair from one-half of his head to enforce seclusion in a cave; filled his mouth with pebbles to correct stuttering; practiced daily before a mirror; copied and recopied the History of Thucydides eight times and committed it to memory; studied under all the great orators of his time and spent eight years in preparing "the greatest oration of the greatest orator of the world."

Lord Brougham allowed himself only four

Manhood's Morning.

hours' sleep. He recopied his greatest speech in the House of Lords twenty times and practiced it for many weeks. Cicero was under constant drill for thirty years and practiced daily before some critic or friend; his life was an incessant drudgery. Pericles never went into the street except to the Forum or Senate and dined out only once during his life. Edmund Burke disclaimed any superior talent. He worked constantly and would have his speeches printed two or three times privately for revision before giving them to the public. It was said of William Pitt that perhaps no man, except Cicero, ever submitted to an equal amount of drudgery. Chesterfield was almost infinite in painstaking and was an indefatigable worker. Lord Chatham went through Bailey's large dictionary twice, carefully studying each word. He translated all the orations of Cicero and practiced daily before a mirror. William Cobbett said: "I have not during my life spent more than thirty-five minutes at table, including all the meals of the day."

Daniel Webster worked twelve hours daily for fifty years. He studied the dictionary almost daily for twenty years. He was an early riser and his classical sentences, now so familiar, were revised over and over again and cost him endless toil. Patrick Henry is reported as being lazy, but the fact remains that he had a

What Young Men Must Do.

large library, was an accomplished Latin and
Greek scholar and studied several hours daily.
Rufus Choate was a slave to the classics and
for forty years not a day passed without an
effort to perfect himself in speech. Henry
Clay made it a rule of his life to talk daily to
the cattle, the cornfields and the woods.
Charles Sumner studied much day and night
all his life. Alexander Hamilton said: "When
I have a subject in hand I study it profoundly.
Day and night it is before me."

John Wesley rose at four, summer and winter; preached twice daily for fifty years and
rode over 270,000 miles during his life. Adam
Clarke spent forty years on his Commentary.
Noah Webster labored for thirty-six years
upon his dictionary and crossed the ocean twice
to gather materials. Gibbon spent twenty-six
years on his "Decline and Fall of the Roman
Empire." Bancroft labored for twenty-six
years on his "History of the United States."
Motley, although a classical literary man, spent
ten years in diligent study before even beginning the history that made him famous. Darwin was not quick to think or write, but his patience and industry were unbounded. He said:
"A man who dares waste one hour of time has
not discovered the value of life." Charles
Dickens was an inveterate slave to hard work.
Milton rose at four in winter and at five in

Manhood's Morning.

summer. Massillon recopied some of his sermons twenty times.

Says Edgar Allan Poe: "Most writers—poets in especial—prefer having it understood that they compose by a species of fine frenzy, an ecstatic intuition; and would positively shudder at letting the public take a peep behind the scenes...—in a word, at the wheels and pinions, the tackle for scene-shifting, the step ladders and demon-traps, the cock's feathers, the red paint and the black patches, which in ninety-nine cases out of the hundred, constitute the properties of the literary *histrio*." Poe is considered America's greatest poetic genius and "The Raven" is his best production; yet of this he himself wrote: "No one point in its composition is referable either to accident or intuition,—the work proceeded step by step to its completion, with the precision and rigid consequence of a mathematical problem."

Virgil labored eleven years on his Æneid and then considered it imperfect. Thomas Gray spent seven years in writing his "Elegy in a Country Church Yard." The fact that Bryant wrote his "Thanatopsis" at the age of eighteen everybody knows; that he revised corrected, transposed and rewrote it no less than one hundred times before giving it to the public is known to but few. Goethe, the German poet and author, was a great genius but a greater prodigy at hard work.

Sir Isaac Newton said: "Whatever service I have done the public was not owing to any extraordinary sagacity, but solely to industry and patient thought." Thomas A. Edison has taken out over seven hundred patents but claims to have made only one discovery through accident. He worked eighteen to twenty hours daily for seven months to perfect the phonograph. He experimented patiently and methodically with 1,800 substances in solving the problem of Roentgen's X rays. His success has been due to "an infinite capacity for taking pains."

The Atlantic cable cost Cyrus W. Field nearly nineteen years of anxious watching and ceaseless toil. He said: "Often my heart has been ready to sink. Many times when wandering in the forests of Newfoundland, in the pelting rain, or on the decks of ships stormy nights alone, far from home, I have almost accused myself of madness and folly." George Stephenson spent fifteen years in perfecting the locomotive. Watt worked for thirty years on the condensing engine. Hard rubber cost Goodyear ten years of study, poverty and ridicule. John Hunter allowed himself only four hours' sleep. Michael Angelo slept in his clothes when engaged in his greatest works and kept food within reach eating a bite at a time. Mendelssohn, Handel and Beethoven were all prodigies at incessant work. No theologian ever labored more diligently than did Benjamin West in evolving his Bible paintings.

There is danger of young men losing the art of work. God has put us here to labor. Before each life stretches its highest possibilities and to reach the summit is the duty of all. Neither genius nor luck alone will prevail. Work must win the race. There are no sinecures in life's highway. Everyone must work with hands, brain and strength. Success is reached by being active, awake, ahead of the crowd; by aiming high, pushing ahead honestly, diligently, patiently; by climbing, digging, saving; by forgetting the past, using the present, trusting in the future; by honoring God, having a purpose, fainting not, determining to win, and striving to the end.

> "Manhood, like gold, is tested in the furnace,
> A fire that purifies is fierce and strong,
> Rare statues gain art's ideal of perfection
> By skillful stroke of chisel wielded long."

Young men must destroy pessimism. Popular opinions regarding life, happiness, success and progress are barnacled with cynical and pessimistic ideas. There is a gloomy, sour impression, almost universal, that the world is as

What Young Men Must Do.

happy and mankind as healthy and prosperous
as God intended they should be; that all the
great men are dead; that the good things are
intended for the few and that the majority of
mankind would not amount to anything under
any conditions. Many believe that

> "Man to misery is born!
> Born to drudge, and sweat and suffer."

Not long since a well known speaker declared that "We cannot expect men of the present day to equal the great masters of the past."
When a good or great man dies we are apt
to believe that

> "He was a man, take him for all in all,
> I shall not look upon his like again,"

thus tacitly acknowledging that the human
race, like the ancient wonders of the world, is
tottering to ruin. Such pessimistic ideas are
a travesty upon manhood and gnaw at the very
vitals of hope, ambition and success.

America will yet lead the world in unfolding God's plans in blessing humanity. The
greatest men are yet to be born and the grandest achievements are yet to be wrought. And
why should it not be so? Has God lost His
omnipotence and His love for the world? Has
mankind buried its genius and talents and

267

Manhood's Morning.

have its hands forgotten their cunning? Have earth's best harvest fields been garnered, its fairest beauties plucked, and its richest treasures absorbed? Is the world's greatest handicraft an ancient ruin? Are its brightest and best men ashes and dust? A thousand times no! The world is yet in its infancy; the glory of a new era is before us; a bright, happy, prosperous age—The Kingdom of God—will surely come.

America is destined to fill a mission and win a greatness distinctively her own. Neither her own proud past nor the trophies of foreign lands can measure her future progress.

It is impossible to perpetuate the eloquence of Demosthenes, Webster, Cicero, Burke, Everett or O'Connell in cold type. But greater orators than these will yet live and their words will inspire the hearts of future generations. Wilberforce, Washington, Jefferson and Adams gave to the nation the principles of liberty, and Lincoln, Phillips, Sumner and Grant have established these principles in the land, but greater statesmen and heroes than these must yet teach liberty to be just and generous, wise and contented.

The names of Hippocrates, Pare, Jenner, Pasteur, Hunter, Rush, Gross and Agnew are written high upon the scroll of fame in Medicine, but physicians will soon live, infinitely more correct in diagnosis and treatment than were these Nestors of their age. Philosophy is proud of the names of Bacon, Socrates, Plato and Franklin, but wisdom greater than they even dreamed is already broadcast over the land. Newton, Young, Comte and Spencer, in the field of Science, and Faraday, Priestley, Berthollet and Davy, in the realm of Chemistry, simply stood upon the first levels of earth's exhaustless mines whose depths shall yet be explored and made subject to man's power and will.

"Earth and Ocean, Flame and Wind
Have unnumbered secrets still,
To be ransacked when you will,
For the service of mankind;
Science is a child as yet,
And her power and scope will grow,
And her triumphs in the future
Shall diminish toil and woe."

The world's best music and poetry belong to the future. The productions of the gifted Haydn, the wonderful Mendelssohn, the magnificent Beethoven and the incomparable Mozart are all exotic to the American ear and climate. Human experiences have been sung in rhyme and metre by Homer, Virgil, Shakespeare, Milton, Tennyson, Burns, Longfellow, Bryant, Lowell, Cowper, Whittier and Holmes, but they echo the past rather than inspire the present or illumine the future. Song and poetry, more than laws, shape history but they must be ahead of, not behind, the times. Every nation and every age require their own song and rhyme. No matter how exquisite and transcendent they may be, time will mar their vital essence. America will yet produce a music and verse of its own, attuned to its own clime, suited to the age that inspires them and cheering the pathway of mankind to the highest summits.

The works of Dickens, Scott, Hugo, Cooper, Hawthorne, Collins, Thackeray, Eliot and Irving are all antiquated and out of date. Their vernacular, and the conditions in which they were plotted have become faded and obscure. Nature needs clothing in new beauties and Nature's heart needs to be touched and quickened by new themes.

Watt, Stephenson, Fulton, Whitney, Howe, Field, Morse, McCormick, Edison and others have revealed a new civilization, yet invention was never so prolific and startling and the future is inconceivably promising.

For four centuries, led by Pestalozzi, Froebel, Jefferson and Horace Mann and a legion of co-workers, education has been climbing up through strata of superstition, error and doubt but it is now ready for a new life. The conquests of learning have scarcely begun but knowledge will yet fill the earth as the waters cover the deep. Even the works of Jesus Christ will be surpassed by those who shall follow after Him. He healed the sick, restored the blind and deaf and dumb; He made the lame to walk and the dead to rise and live again. Yet it was He who said: "He that believeth on Me the works that I do he shall do also, and greater works than these shall he do."

Future progress will represent the masses rather than the few. "It seems very certain," says Phillips Brooks, "that the world is to grow better and richer in the future, * * * not by the magnificent achievements of the highly gifted few, but by the patient faithfulness of the one-talented many." More reciprocal and diffused conditions between the gifted and less favored are destined to prevail. The parable of the talents not only shows the intimate relation between the gifted and ordinary, but also that the five talented *can* and the one talented *must* fulfill their mission. All classes will recognize the common brotherhood, all will aid the common good and all will secure a deserved share of success.

Young men must endure and transcend fogyism. The world is as full of fogyism as water is of microbes and there are a million in every drop. Fogyism is the self-imposed jury which

271

Manhood's Morning.

sits in judgment and, without even a mock trial, condemns and pronounces sentence upon its victims. It is as old as sin and resembles it closely. It has followed civilization from the beginning and is alive and lusty as ever. For sixty centuries it has cried: "It won't work." "It can't be done." "Let good enough alone." "I told you so"—free to all. From the moss-covered heights of self-content it sings:

> "Stand ye still! ye restless nations,
> And be happy where you are,
> Change is rash and never wise
> If ye meddle we will mar."

Fogyism has ridiculed, scoffed, pooh-poohed, hissed and persecuted almost every good man and every improvement since the world began. No penalty is too base for its prejudice, no missile is too vile for its hate. It will fire anathemas from the pulpit or wrath from the platform; it will hurl calumny from the pew or rotten eggs from the mob.

> "Truths would you teach to save a sinking land,
> All fear, none aid you, and few understand."

Long before the rivers were channels of commerce they served to protect new nations from old enemies; mountains have simply been fences to separate fogyisms too desperate to live neighbors; oceans have been too narrow to insure safe lands of refuge to men with thoughts and opinions of their own.

Galileo, after inventing the clock pendulum, the telescope, and devoting his life for others, was forced to bow his venerable head, whitened by seventy winters, and "abjure, curse and detest the aforesaid errors and heresies." Old and blind and imprisoned, he exclaimed: "My name is erased from the book of the living." "The Revolution of the Celestial Orbs," cost Copernicus twenty-two years of labor but he dared not publish it. Roger Bacon was persecuted for his wisdom, accused of magic; his books were burned in public, and he was imprisoned for ten years.

For conceiving steam navigation, DeCaus was pronounced insane and thrown into the mad-house. When John Fitch invented a steamboat, the public, not even Franklin, would notice it. He sat down and wrote: "Some more powerful man will get fame and riches from my invention" and then committed suicide. Robert Fulton tells us that during the entire time he was building his steamboat: *"Never did a single encouraging remark, a bright hope or a warm wish cross my path."*

The steam engine cost Watt almost martyrdom. He said: "The struggles I have had with natural difficulties and with ignorance,

Manhood's Morning.

prejudices and villainies of mankind, have been very great. * * * There is nothing more foolish than inventing." Rapid locomotion was strongly condemned. Riding rapidly "would injure people." "They would swallow wind;" "lose their breath." "The cattle would be frightened to death," and Parliament was requested to limit speed to nine miles an hour. United States Chancellor Livingston wrote an article proving railroads utterly impossible.

The use of gas was ridiculed by the great chemist, Davy, and Wollaston, the scientist, said: "They might as well attempt to use a slice out of the moon."

Demonstrating the circulation of the blood cost Dr. Harvey many of his patients and the physicians violently assailed him, not one over forty years old admitting the truth of his discovery. Vaccination cost Jenner sixteen years experimenting and vehement opposition; societies being started and journals printed to oppose it. The eminent discoverer, Priestly, had his house pillaged, its contents burned by a mob and he was forced to flee from his country.

Columbus encountered incessant ridicule and opposition. His crew assailed him to the verge of mutiny, he was chained on board his own ship, imprisoned by his own countrymen and died poor, neglected and broken-hearted.

Charles V. in an edict said: "No one shall print, write, copy, keep, conceal, sell, buy, or give any book written by Martin Luther, or any other heretic." Another edict read: "All heretics shall be put to death." The churches were closed against John Wesley and on several occasions he had to flee for his life. Fox, the founder of the Society of Friends, was imprisoned. William Penn, a prominent member, was disowned by his parents, ostracised and sent to jail; a clergyman wrote a book against the sect under the rancorous title of "Hell Let Loose." Sunday-schools were at first opposed. When Miss Lathrop started one in Connecticut it was turned out of the church, then out of the school house, then out of the court house; but she kept on and in fifty years this school had sent out twenty-six ministers and hundreds of Christian workers; H. P. Haven, "The Model Superintendent," being, as a small boy, a charter scholar.

Fogyism has always opposed liberty and independence. When the colonists declared for liberty and said: "We mutually pledge to each other our lives, our fortunes and our sacred honor," it aroused the most intense antagonism of the most powerful nation in the world. Triumph over slavery in England cost Wilber-

Manhood's Morning.

force nineteen years of "slander, insult, bitterness of hope deferred, the coldness and treachery of friends and the persistent malice of enemies." Freedom in America made Wendell Phillips "as an outcast * * * deserted and avoided, as though stricken with the leprosy;" it made Garrison a prisoner, a scapegoat and a target for the mob; it cost Lincoln martyrdom and the Nation the life's blood of hundreds of thousands of its noblest and bravest men.

Were it not for young men progressive enterprise would almost cease. The old, as a rule, are skeptical and oppose new ideas. Every generation and every life develops a new history.

> "New occasions teach new duties;
> Time makes ancient good uncouth;
> They must upward, still, and onward,
> Who would keep abreast of Truth.
> Lo! before us gleam her camp-fires!
> We, ourselves, must Pilgrims be.
> Launch our Mayflower, and steer boldly
> Through the desperate winter sea.
> Nor attempt the Future's portal
> With the Past's blood-rusted key."

Difficulties and oppositions develop the heroic in young men. But for the husks the prodigal would never have feasted on fatted calf. Hisses from the crowd kindled the fires

of eloquence in Demosthenes. "O, what a
stupid ass!" from his teacher turned a lazy
boy into Adam Clarke. The ridicule and sar-
casm of Parliament made Disraeli the greatest
man in England. Bitter opposition was an
inspiration to Martin Luther; the more angry
he was the more zealously could he preach,
pray and work. Bedford Jail and Bunyan
wrote "Pilgrims' Progress"; neither could do
it alone. "There is no possible success," said
Dr. Holmes, without some opposition as a ful-
crum."

Men are not roused into action by recom-
pense, pleasures, hope of ease, or sugar-plums
of any sort, but by trials, abnegation, hardships and even martyrdom. Adversity awak-
ens talent; the greater the obstacles the more
earnest the zeal; the stronger the opposition
the more heroic and determined is the life of
the true man.

*Young men must perfect the health and
physique of the race.* Young men only can
do this. From two to five generations of pure,
undefiled manhood would produce a race without an inherited blemish. America will never
be great or good, strong or wise until its people are pure blooded, pure brained and healthy.
Every fireside is interested in this subject.
"Come, let us live for our children," said the
great teacher, Froebel. "Begin to train your

Manhood's Morning.

children twenty years before they are born,"
said the poet-physician, Holmes. Too much
stress is placed upon motherhood, and not
enough upon the fatherhood of posterity. Sentiment demands pure mothers, but God demands pure fathers. It is the "sins of the
fathers" which blight the children. It is when
the fathers eat "sour grapes" that the teeth
of the children are "set on edge." "The glory
of a child is its father," said Solomon. Nothing counts for more than a reliable pedigree,
and nowhere is it more consistent in its mani-
festations than in our children. Most children
are like their parents—*only more so.*

The utmost effort is being made to improve
the stock, species, or varieties among animals,
fruits, vegetables and flowers, and why not give
as much attention to the improvement and perfection of the highest type of creation—man?
It is as essential that the people be taught to
know and respect the laws concerning heredity, as those referring to political economy.
It is as important to know how to preserve
good health and prevent disease, as it is to
master some craft whereby to secure food,
clothing and shelter.

It is for young men, and not for the doctors,
to drive disease, pain, deformity and premature
death from the land. Every child born healthy
proves that all may, accidents excepted, be so

What Young Men Must Do.

blessed, and such will be the case when the bodies of young men become the temples of purity that God intended that they should be. The race will not suffer sickness, pain and deformity any longer than they are necessary and self-inflicted.

Young men can decree that there shall be no more consumption, scrofula, specific ulcers, cancers, loathsome catarrh, insanity and imbecility; no diseases too vile to mention—no wicked and hellish hereditary blush stamped upon a daughter's cheek, and no alluring and suggestive twinkle in her eye; no inherited appetites to weaken the will of a son and no father's sin to drag him down to ruin.

Too little attention is paid to physical development. Religion excepted, health is the highest concern. Indeed, religion and health are wedded virtues. Much of the sin in the world is disease and much of the religion we meet is good health. Health is the vital principle of bliss and the chief source of success. A healthy stomach and a liver that never complains render a man, not only happy, but forceful and invulnerable. No seriously defective young man should ever marry, and there should be laws regulating such marriages. An era of common sense and conscience should supplant prevailing sentimentalisms in love affairs. The time has come when, not only

279

Manhood's Morning.

health, but the sensibilities, faculties and character are born rather than acquired—when all are severely tested and tried and only the fittest survive.

Pure blood should paint the cheeks, and an upright fatherhood should inspire the heart of every boy and girl born upon American soil. It is criminal for young men to flagrantly ignore these subjects as they do. It is the duty of young men to become the fathers of an improved race—of children inheriting all the advantages of healthful vigor; strong in muscle and elastic in limb, clear of eye and magnetic of expression, symmetrical in faculties and temperament, modest in manners and cultured in habits; with minds sound and well poised and with wills kindly set but invincible as steel.

> "Nor love nor honor, wealth nor power,
> Can give the heart a cheerful hour,
> When HEALTH is lost. Be timely wise;
> With HEALTH all taste of pleasure flies."

Young men must destroy ignorance. As a cause of misery, degradation and unhappiness, ignorance stands first. It is more destructive than poverty or disease, and ruins more lives than temptation and willfulness combined. Through lack of knowledge the people perish. Next to sin, ignorance is the world's curse.

What Young Men Must Do.

Squalor, sickness and premature death are little else than the fruits of ignorance. According to statistics, ignorance, in the form of incompetency and inexperience, causes more failures in business than extravagance, neglect, competition, speculation, fraud and unwise credit combined. And what is true in the matter of business is still more true in professional life and in the realm of labor. Ignorance is darkness, weakness, failure and ruin, while knowledge is light, strength, success, opportunity and life. Ignorance is God's worst enemy and Satan's best friend. And to none is ignorance so great a curse, and to none is knowledge so great a boon as to young men. It is the duty of every one to thoroughly detest ignorance.

The progress and success of the future will be intellectual. Education, culture, science, art, ethics and refinement will create and establish demand and supply. There is no knowledge that is not power. Progress is simply more light. A foolish notion exists that "the world is growing weaker and wiser." Such a thing is impossible; only ignorance can impair; genuine wisdom always improves, edifies and constructs.

Ignorance is a chief cause of business depressions and hard times. The labor, financial and other political and social questions are

Manhood's Morning.

largely battles between ignorance and knowledge. Nothing will bring substantial and permanent prosperity so surely as the spread of
education and culture. Indeed, there is no
other way to establish permanent and genuine
thrift. Only as knowledge, in its broadest and
best sense, increases, will the capacity to desire
and enjoy and the ability to produce multiply.

The demand for intellectual workers is
boundless and will never be fully supplied,
while the demand for manual labor is limited
and constantly growing less. With new
knowledge come new abilities and powers,
new comforts and new necessities. As a rule,
it is easier for an enlarged mind to secure its
increased desires than for a benighted, aimless
intellect to obtain its bare necessities. Labor,
to the former, is strength and development, to
the latter, compulsory drudgery.

To multiply desires, comforts and necessities,
and make it possible for all to secure them, is a
potent factor in civilization and enlightenment.
Intellectual needs are infinitely more prolific
than physical needs; indeed, *more knowledge*
is "Nature's Remedy" for over production
and idle men and mills. God and Nature provide abundantly everywhere, and in nothing
are they so liberal as when contributing to the
comforts and desires of mankind. It is not
genuine Christian discipline to needlessly deny

ourselves any good thing. Excessive economy in the use of that which is good for us will never bring prosperity. Stinginess can only stop the wheels of enterprise. The close-fisted miser is usually a social vagabond, if not an infidel. God wants all his children to enjoy far more of the good things around them than they are ready to believe or admit.

Not only does knowledge increase desires and the ability to gratify these desires, but it makes men more aesthetic, refined and discriminating. It creates a demand for a better standard of quality. To know of a good thing is to want it. To understand quality causes a demand for the best. Mankind will never do itself justice until it secures everything it needs, and until all these things are the best that human skill, industry and genius can produce.

As ignorance is destroyed and knowledge increases, supply and demand will undergo a revolution. With improved intellectual conceptions the people will demand better clothes and houses, better markets and harvests, better milk and butter, bread and beefsteak, better horses and cattle, farms and farmers, fruits and flowers, better roads and methods of locomotion, better newspapers and books, teachers and leaders, better doctors and medicine, better manhood and morals, mind and manners, better fathers and mothers, husbands and wives, sons and daughters, better churches and creeds, preachers and Christians, better laws and lawyers, officials and citizens, better work and better pay, better employers and employes, better homes and better hearts, better hopes and better joys. The millennium will be little else than that good time when knowledge shall fill the earth, and when every human need will be met and when every man will be liberally supplied from the abundance.

Young men must destroy poverty. There is a poverty in our nation constantly growing more widespread and organic, which is slavish, unjust and oppressive. It is too true that poverty has become the menace of all and the inevitable doom of a vast number. Our nation during four centuries has accumulated property to the value of nearly $100,000,000,000. But in dealing it out to her children, practically the whole amount has been given to one million men, leaving over sixty million with only a pittance. Seventy per cent. of the wealth of the nation has been given to 200,000 men. Each one of these men, on an average, hold enough possessions, either active or latent, to support one thousand of his neighbors and, at the same time, a majority of these neighbors are struggling against poverty and must live and die poor in spite of themselves.

Not only is the wealth in the hands of a few,

What Young Men Must Do.

but we are fostering a system of industrial bondage. Said Hon. H. A. Herbert, formerly Secretary of the Navy, in a recent address: "We are entering upon an era of vast enterprises that threaten to occupy, to the exclusion of others, all the avenues of human progress." Capitalized corporations, gigantic enterprises, mammoth stores, railroads reaching from lakes to gulf, or from ocean to ocean, under one management, industrial plants with millions of capital, protected by trusts, combinations and law, are rapidly taking possession of the field and smaller enterprises are destined to disappear. "Human wit," says Mr. Herbert, "seems unable to devise, without dangerously curtailing the natural liberty of the citizen, any plan for the prevention of these monopolies, and the effect is the accumulation of vast wealth by the few and the narrowing opportunities of the many."

The love of money is the master passion of the American people. Wealth is our aristocracy; it rules in politics, makes our laws and is the octopus in manufacturing and commerce. Wealth has grown aggressive, heartless and over-powering, while poverty has become embarrassed, passive and weak. Even honest toil —the curse of honest sweat—at fair wages has become a luxury that is denied to many. There are multitudes of men and women, represent-

285

ing the choice fibre of the race, who are as veritable slaves to the sordid demands of wealth as were the human chattels that hoed the corn and picked the cotton in the "Sunny South" in "Sixty-one." In form of government we are a republic, in practical experience we are a despotism; in religion we are Christians, in business we are cannibals.

Nothing is more certain than that the inherited and legitimate road to life, liberty and the pursuit of happiness is being narrowed and obstructed by the power of concentrated wealth. It is also true that no people are so embarrassed and humiliated by poverty as Americans; and in no land is poverty so unnecessary, so out of place or so abominable as in the United States.

"Wealth in the dross is death, but life diffused;
As poison heals, in just proportions used;
In heap, like ambergris, a stink it lies,
But, well dispersed, is incense to the skies.

"The danger," said Dr. Howard Crosby, "which threatens the uprooting of society, the demolition of civil institutions, the destruction of liberty, and the desolation of all, is that which comes from the rich and powerful classes in the community." At a time when Benjamin Harrison had cause to ponder well his words he said: "I do not believe that a republic can live and prosper whose wage-earners do not receive enough to make life comfortable; who do not have some upward avenue of hope before them."

America is the richest nation on earth, and its rapid development and increase of wealth have no parallel. Above a livelihood, we are increasing in riches $3,000,000,000 annually, or over $7,000,000 daily; more than $2,000 for every boy that becomes a man. Our nation is capable of supporting 1,000,000,000 people, and its present population could be supported by four of its largest States, leaving forty States unoccupied. It might be said that the sun never sets upon our possessions; before his last rays fade from the western isles of Alaska the dawning sunlight falls upon the pines of Maine.

In such a nation there should be a constant and inexhaustible demand for young men. There should be abundant room for all, work for every pair of hands and a just reward for every honest effort. It should be possible for every young man to, not only earn a livelihood, but to develop and accumulate and, at a proper time get married under favorable prospects, to support his family and rear his children respectably, to build a home and eventually pay for it, to furnish it with all the comforts of modern convenience, to supply the library with the best of books and the centre-table with the best of magazines, to keep all comfortably and

Manhood's Morning.

even fashionably clothed, both summer and winter; to live upon seasonable, wholesome food, to secure good educational and church advantages, to afford time for recreation, entertainments and amusements, to keep coal in the bin, credit in the community and money in the bank, to have much to enjoy and more to love and to retire at a proper season and enjoy his declining years as a reward for his labors.

The development of the home-life to its full and proper extent would obliterate hard times forever. Millions of homes should be built at once and enough furniture, household goods, cooking utensils, pianos, books, paintings, and useful and beautiful commodities are needed to keep every factory running day and night, and every hand and brain, every artist and artisan busy for a decade. The universal ownership of homes is the palladium of national safety and contentment. Then will men have something to love and cherish; then will the financial and industrial questions settle themselves. Every young man should be taught to look forward to a home of his own, to pray for it, to strive for it, and, if necessary, fight for it.

Poverty, as it exists to-day, is a concrete wrong. It is the mother of crime and the chief cause of intemperance, ignorance and degradation. That the rich are growing more wealthy and more fortified in their possessions, and the

288

poor more dependent and doomed is a disgrace as shameful as it is momentous.

Poverty is chiefly a political condition. While it is reached by a thousand paths and while much of that which exists shows individual faults, yet existing conditions are such as to strongly favor poverty and make it the unavoidable lot of multitudes of people. It will never be overthrown or greatly lessened until it is done through political action.

It is unmistakably true that the destruction of poverty means that the many, instead of the few, must control the wealth of the nation. So long as extreme wealth is possible and desirable to a few, extreme poverty will be the enforced fate of the many. So long as America is the paradise of the rich it will be the purgatory of the poor.

With rare exceptions, concentrated wealth is unscrupulous, heartless and despotic. "The love of money is the root of all evil." The nation is crowded with men who worship at the shrine of greed; mammon is their god; they "will be rich," and to obtain their goal are willing to resort to methods "which drown men in destruction and perdition." "Avarice and luxury have been the ruin of every State." May it never be said of America that poverty

"Crushes into dumb despair
One-half the human race."

Manhood's Morning.

When wealth, in the power of its concentration, monopolizes and oppresses, corners and crushes; when it grows sordid, heartless and despotic; when it brings starvation, rags and ignorance; when it breeds slaves, paupers and criminals; when it becomes un-American and unjust; when it hedges our pathway with man-traps and temptations, and plays upon our passions and credulity as strategems of business; when it debases politics, pollutes morals, defies law, obliterates the Sabbath and corrupts literature; when it disgraces the face of the nation with haunts of shame and dram-shops that ruin one hundred daughters and bury in dishonored graves two hundred sons, every day in the year; when it ceases to be a blessing to those who hold it or a benefit to others, then it becames a common foe and a national peril, to be hated, controlled and scattered. For young men to ignore their responsibility under such conditions is political and religious perfidy, cowardice and treason.

It is not possible for political isms or political demagogues, hungry for the spoils of office, to lessen poverty. These are morbid growths upon the body politic and are, of themselves, evils to be routed and destroyed. The rich will never antagonize poverty, and their benefactions, no matter how princely, can never atone for its cause. Help and philanthropy

What Young Men Must Do.

cannot substitute inherited rights. It dwarfs manhood to trail as the protege and puppet of wealth. "Nine-tenths of the money given to benefit the healthy poor does more harm than good." Nor can gigantic industries improve existing conditions. A century ago Franklin said: "The time will come when men will not have to work more than four or five hours daily to meet the demands of labor." Labor-saving machinery and business combinations are making his prophecy true. Human wit was never more anxious to curtail expenses, invent machines to do the work of men, to concentrate force and labor and send men adrift in idleness. Mankind must learn to look elsewhere than to the rich or to wage-earning for occupation and success in life.

Young men have the inherited right, the essential strength and the patriotic incentives to overthrow poverty and drive it from the land. The conflict is theirs and it belongs to none other. Over three million young men vote for the first time at each national election. They are not simply the "balance of power" but they are the power itself. Every vote of theirs should go to crush a wrong and free a righteous cause and make that cause enthroned.

Young men have no right to remain passive and consign themselves to poverty's enslaving and degrading influence and their families to a

Manhood's Morning.

life-long struggle against privation. "He who fails to provide for his own house," writes the Apostle, "denies the faith and is worse than an infidel." "He that despiseth the gain of oppressions," says the Prophet, "bread shall be given him." No matter what brings poverty to our doors it should be feared, hated and assailed as desperately as would be a savage wolf that seeks to invade our firesides and steal our children.

It is the duty of young men to demand that life's pathway reach down to the level of the lowest and, unobstructed and broad enough for all, reach the summit of the highest possibilities. Wealth should be the servant of all mankind and the master of none. It should be support to the weak, power to the worthy and a loyal and potent force in building the nation. Wealth should make it possible for all to honorably succeed and unnecessary for any to wholly fail. Wealth should be the possession of the people and poverty, in free America, should be unknown.

Young men must forward and exalt the nation. Great is the work of Americans. We are entering upon an era of the world's history surpassing beyond comparison, any past age.

> "We are living, we are dwelling
> In a grand and awful time,
> In an age on ages telling
> To be living is sublime!"

What Young Men Must Do.

Confidence in the future has become a part of the national faith. Never did the people so quickly absorb and implicitly trust in new ideas and inventions. Genius and talent no longer live and die unappreciated. A market is always in waiting for the product of the most gifted brain or the more skillful hand. The people accept with unbounded confidence every worthy contribution to the world's greatness.

Mechanical invention is so rapid that it is revolutionary in its effects. In electricity, alone, there are, in the United States of America, 1,000,000 miles of telegraph, by which are sent 65,000,000 messages annually, and there are in operation several millions telephones. "Electricity," says Chauncey Depew, "is to be largely the substitute for the horse; . . . it is to furnish light for dwelling and factory, for hospital and highway; it is to give heat for cooking and for comfort; it is to be the power for the machinery of mill and the press of newspaper; it is to be the motor for transportation by land and sea." From the coal mines come not only heat, light and power, but any color, from printer's ink to the tint of the rarest flower; any flavor, from the strawberry or peach to the substance, saccharine, two hundred times sweeter than sugar; and from coal, science has evolved remedies that will cool the fevered brow and modify the bounding pulse,

Manhood's Morning.

soothe the excited nerves and bring quiet and refreshing sleep. Never were the hidden and priceless treasures of earth so rapidly discovered and transformed into utility as now. New uses for air, water, and the elements of nature follow each other in rapid succession. Niagara has entered upon a multiform mission of usefulness, and is driving the wheels of industry, turning darkness into light and carrying mankind to and fro by transmitted power. All nature, it would seem, has become enchanted and is offering itself as a sacrifice in man's behalf, and, with startling possibilities and magic powers, is following his bidding.

And we will not stop in our onward march. For a decade the advent of a "New South," the costliest possession that adorns our national domain, has led in a general transformation. In the great West a cluster of new States have won a place upon the American ensign. The North and East have ceased to glory in their age and, with renewed and more youthful vigor, are awakening to a more enterprising spirit. The cities and towns have caught the inspiration and a *new* and greater New York, a *new* and more substantial Chicago and a *new* and more modern Philadelphia pass the watchword to smaller cities, towns and hamlets until with renewed zeal and energy, the nation is filled with industry, bustle and enterprise.

What Young Men Must Do.

Politics is feeling the force of improvement. Antiquated notions and fossilized issues are ceasing to command support, and the questions and issues of the new age are demanding the attention of patriotic and thoughtful men.

The Church is renewing her youth, and, like a bride clad in wedding garments, she is inviting the young and vigorous to her sanctuaries. "Lift up your eyes," says an eminent writer, "and you may see another stadium of history advancing. Its aim will be to realize the Christianity of Christ Himself, which is about to renew its youth by taking to heart the Sermon on the Mount. He that sitteth on the throne is saying: *'Behold I make all things new.'* This earth is yet to be redeemed, soul and body with all its peoples, occupations and interests.'" Glorious thought! Wonderful consummation! Blessed is he who helps!

All about us are the inspiring awakenings of a new century—the beginning of another thousand years. The progress of the past and the activity of the present will add momentum to the future and it is unspeakably full of promise. "The future is lighted up for us," says John Fiske, "with the radiant colors of hope. Strife and sorrow will disappear. Peace and love shall reign supreme. The dream of the poets, the lesson of the priest and prophet, the inspiration of the great musician, is con-

Manhood's Morning.

firmed in the light of modern knowledge." Let us believe that man will yet banish the darkness of night and overcome the sting of the winter's cold and the oppression of the summer's sun; that he will penetrate the mysteries of space and look through the clouded abyss of time; that he will destroy ignorance, oppression, disease, wickedness and subdue the earth unto himself. When man exercises his divinely intended dominion over the kingdoms of nature, the earth in homage will blossom and bloom and bear fruit as a tribute to human industry, intelligence and virtue.

The United States is the chosen home of the Anglo-Saxon race—the race of virtue, liberty and progress. This race, which America is destined to develop to the highest perfection, has, for twelve centuries, been gaining conquests, growing in influence and in civilization until it has become the unrivalled and dominating race of the earth.

America has become a World Power. In 1700 the Anglo-Saxons numbered less than 6,000,000 souls, while, at the present time, there are over 120,000,000. They have increased more than five-fold during the present century and are multiplying more rapidly than all the races of continental Europe combined, and it is possible that by the end of another century they will outnumber all the civilized nations of the earth.

They are the most powerful and the richest nation in the world. They are in possession of one-third of the earth and rule over not less than 400,000,000 people. They own sixty per cent. of the railroads, more than one-half the telegraphs and two-thirds of the world's shipping. The time is not far distant when this one race will hold more than one-half of the wealth of the globe.

The Anglo-Saxons are the greatest law-making and the most systematic people in the world, and they have a genius for organization. They framed the Magna Charta of Great Britain, "the first popular basis of human liberty," the Declaration of Independence and the Constitution of the United States, which Gladstone declared to be "the most wonderful work ever struck off at a given time by the brain or purpose of man." This race enjoys nearly all the civil liberty in the world. Its battles have been for worthy principles, and its conquests have been victories for liberty, justice and truth.

The Anglo-Saxon is the Christian nation of the world. Its religion is the religion of The Bible, its God is the Lord and its faith is in the Risen Christ. It is the race of heroes, martyrs, statesmen, poets, philosophers, scientists, inventors, scholars and benefactors. It has in-

Manhood's Morning.

vented steam-power, railroads, steam navigation, telegraphs, the improved printing press,
the use of ether, the sewing machine, cotton
gin, spinning jenny and harvesting machine;
the value of coal, illuminating gas and the
power of electricity.

The Anglo-Saxon race has always been the
champion and exemplar of high social standards. While yet barbarians in the German
wilds, the fathers and founders of the race were
"as pure as the dews the forests shook upon
their heads." Roman historians state that
"The adulterer was buried alive in the mud, and
the adulteress was publicly whipped through
the streets." "Non forma, non aetate, non
opibus maritum invenerit." Out of this race
sprang Chivalry and for a thousand years it
has taken the lead in high moral reforms and a
pure family life. Its political, social and religious history has been marked by great moral
uplifts. Beginning with the Reformation and
Protestantism, Methodism, Presbyterianism,
Quakerism, Puritanism, Sunday-schools, the
Temperance Crusade, the Young Men's Christian Association, the Woman's Christian Temperance Union, the Salvation Army and the
Young People's Society of Christian Endeavor
have been organized efforts for a higher and
cleaner life, and, with one exception, all of
these were of Anglo-Saxon origin.

What Young Men Must Do.

The two great divisions of the Anglo-Saxon race, Great Britain and the United States, are the most enlightened, powerful and progressive nations in the world, and more than one-half of the race live in the United States. The United States is richer, more energetic and progressive than Great Britain, and is more Anglo-Saxon than English in its genius and typical characteristics. Evidently the North American Continent is destined to become the future home of the highest expression of this great race.

The United States, to a remarkable degree, is adapted to such a people. In climate, productiveness of soil, wealth of mine, water power, rivers and geographical and natural advantages, nature has been, not only abundant, but lavish.

In climate, the United States is almost perfect. Spring, summer, autumn and winter are well developed, but none are so severe or prolonged as to prove debilitating or monotonous. Rain and sunshine, storm and calm, wind and zephyr, succeed each other and form an interesting panorama, and the weather is always a welcome subject for comment. Our agricultural resources are beyond calculation. We grow the kings of human sustenance. Our wheat and corn, fruit and cotton, cattle and horses, sheep and hogs, on account of their abundance and perfection, are sought by the markets of the world. In manufacturing we are developing an era peculiarly our own. Abundance of materials, inventive genius and diligent enterprise are sending civilizing products to every corner of the globe.

Our language is the most flexible, forceful, direct and powerful the world has produced. It is the language of Chaucer, Shakespeare, Milton, Burns, Dryden, Addison, Wordsworth, Macaulay, Scott, Dickens, Tennyson, Erskine, Pitt, O'Connell, Wilberforce, Johnson, Livingstone, Stanley, Gladstone and every American statesman, writer, poet, inventor and teacher. It is the dominating language of the world, to-day. Enshrined in its embrace are Liberty, Law, Love and the message of Eternal Life.

The Anglo-Saxon language, of which our nation furnishes the highest expression, is better fitted than any other to become the language of the world. Its power to assimilate and expand is unlimited. Says Dr. Schaff: "Its composite character imparts to it a pliability, expansiveness and perfectability which no other language possesses;" and in the opinion of Dr. Grimm, the eminent philologist, "in wealth, intellectuality and closeness of structure, none of all the living languages can be compared with it."

300

What Young Men Must Do.

The United States is not only ahead of any other nation, but none is achieving so much or advancing so rapidly. "Ten years in America," says a noted Englishman, "is half a century of European progress," and our rate of speed is rapidly, even amazingly, on the increase.

It is self-evident that God designated the United States as the Model Republic and the great evangelizer of the world. The discovery of America was the greatest triumph of civilization. "Our whole history," says Emerson, "seems like a last effort of the Divine Providence in behalf of the human race." "The Americans," says Herbert Spencer, "may reasonably look forward to a time when they will have produced a civilization grander than the world has known."

The eyes of all lands are upon our own. America is the leader, the teacher, the exemplar of the world. Her two evangels are civil and religious liberty, and these must be lifted high to maintain an honored and glorious career. She must lay aside the implements of battle and blood and go forth arrayed in the emblems of peace. To be as good as our fathers we must be better; to serve our generation as well as they did theirs we must be stronger and wiser. The prophecy of Sumner has come to pass: "The national example is more puissant than army or navy for the conquest of the world."

The chief factor in all these harvests of wealth and upward and onward movements, have been, and must continue to be, the young men of the nation. They are the heirs and owners of a sacred and proud inheritance. It is for them to accept it, to honor, amplify and uphold it and hand it down, even more rich in fruitage, to their children.

As it has been in war so it must be in the grandeurs and glories of peace, young men must do the work. A noble ancestry admonishes them and the world turns to them with solicitous eyes. Only by morality, by industry, by patriotism, by religion and by the cultivation of every righteous principle and every good habit can they fill their lofty mission and transmit, unimpaired, the tenures and triumphs of the nation.

INDEX.

303

307

What is said of Manhood's Morning

From FRANCES E. WILLARD, President National W. C. T. U.

MANHOOD'S MORNING is as far from namby-pamby as a book can be. Dr. Conwell has read widely and thought profoundly. He is also warm-blooded and sympathetic; indeed he seems to have all the characteristics essential to the writing of a helpful book for young men. * * * We advise parents to send for it, giving it as a birthday present to their sons.

Rev. M. L. HAINES, First Presbyterian Church, Indianapolis, Ind. (Ex-President Harrison's Pastor.)

Any parent or friend desirous of conferring a valuable gift upon a young man can do so by presenting him with a copy of MANHOOD'S MORNING. It is a fresh and stimulating book and deals in a practical and common sense way with the problems of a young man's life in our time. The author holds up high ideals and sets forth clearly and convincingly, facts that are of the largest importance in the making of manhood.

Hon. ELI F. RITTER, the eminent Lawyer and Statesman of Indiana.

MANHOOD'S MORNING is a book which has evidently been prepared with great care and research. It bears the impress on every page of the highest motive by its author. If every young man in the land could be induced to read and study it, it would make a great impression for his good. I take pleasure in commending this book especially to young men and to parents who have the responsibility of their training.

MARY WOOD-ALLEN, M. D., Ann Arbor, Mich., Author and Editor *"The New Crusade."*

I have given MANHOOD'S MORNING quite a thorough examination and like it much. It is inspiring and elevating and must be ennobling in its influence. You have done a good work for young men and I thank you for it.

T. J. SANDERS, A. M., Ph. D., President Otterbein University, Ohio.

MANHOOD'S MORNING is carefully and ably written. The book consists of a remarkable series of chapters to young men. They will be very stimulating and suggestive. It will surely do good. I wish all young men could read it.

Prof. F. W. STELLHORN, President Capital University, Columbus, Ohio.

Whilst I cannot adopt every single view found in MAN-HOOD'S MORNING, I am glad to be able to say that it is an exceedingly interesting and instructive book. It may some-times seem to exaggerate a little the relative importance of young men * * * but it cannot but do good wherever it goes. God bless the book, its author, and its readers.

Rev. W. O. FRIES, Westerville, Ohio.

MANHOOD'S MORNING is just such a book as every young man should read. Parents can make no better investment for their sons than this book. Young men should purchase it if they have to go hungry by missing a meal. It is an in-spiration.

Rev. AUSTIN HUNTER, Washington, Ohio.

I have just finished reading MANHOOD'S MORNING. The book is great. I recommend it to young and old ones also. I predict for it a large sale.

W. G. HANNA, in *Mail-Empire*, Toronto, Canada.

MANHOOD'S MORNING exactly meets the case. The title represents the theme exactly. It is far and away, the best book that has yet appeared on the subject. A copy should be in the hands of every young man in Canada.

"What a Young Boy Ought to Know"

For Boys under Sixteen Years of Age

WHAT EMINENT PEOPLE SAY

Theodore L. Cuyler, D.D.

" 'What a Young Boy Ought to Know' ought to be in every home where there is a boy."

Lady Henry Somerset

"Calculated to do an immense amount of good. I sincerely hope it may find its way to many homes."

Joseph Cook, D.D., LL.D.

"It is everywhere suggestive, inspiring and strategic in a degree, as I think, not hitherto matched in literature of its class."

Charles L. Thompson, D.D.

"Why was not this book written centuries ago?"

Anthony Comstock

"It lifts the mind and thoughts upon a high and lofty plane upon delicate subjects."

Edward W. Bok

"It has appealed to me in a way which no other book of its kind has."

Bishop John H. Vincent, D.D., LL.D.

"You have handled with great delicacy and wisdom an exceedingly difficult subject."

John Willis Baer

"I feel confident that it can do great good, and I mean that my boys shall have the contents placed before them."

Mrs. Mary A. Livermore, LL.D.

"Full of physiological truths, which all children ought to know, at a proper age; will be read by boys without awakening a prurient thought."

Josiah Strong, D.D.

"A foolish and culpable silence on the part of most parents leaves their children to learn, too often from vicious companions, sacred truth in an unhallowed way."

"What a Young Man Ought to Know."

BY SYLVANUS STALL, D. D.

Condensed Table of Contents

Price $\left\{ \begin{matrix} \$1.00 \\ 4 \text{ s.} \end{matrix} \right\}$ net, per copy, post free

"What a Young Man Ought to Know."

Commendations of *"Young Man"—Continued.*

The Right Rev. William N. McVickar, D. D.

"I heartily endorse and recommend 'What a Young Man ought to Know.' I believe that it strikes at the very root of matters, and ought to be instrumental for much good."

Ethelbert D. Warfield, I L. D.

"The subject is one of the utmost personal and social importance, and hitherto has not been treated, so far as I am aware, in such a way as to merit the commendation of the Christian public."

Frank W. Ober.

"I have not only carefully examined the book myself, but have submitted it to a competent physician, who has for years received the freest confidence of young men. I take pleasure in commending the book heartily and unqualifiedly to young men. It will save many a young fellow from the blast and blight of a befouled manhood, wrecked by the wretched blunderings of an ignorant youth."

Frederick Anthony Atkins.

"Such books as yours have long been needed, and if they had appeared sooner many a social wreck, whose fall was due to ignorance, might have been saved."

PRESS NOTICES.

"One of the best treatises of the sort ever published."—Congregationalist.

"In these books Dr. Stall has done a service for the cause of humanity, the cause of purity and righteousness among men, which cannot be overestimated."—Christian Work.

"Will save multitudes of men from the paths of vice and ruin."—Christian Advocate.

"The author is very frank, but in dealing with the delicate phases of his subject he is eminently considerate, and shows consummate good taste."—Cumberland Presbyterian.

"The book will be a true and helpful friend to multitudes of young women."—The Christian Endeavor World.

"What a Young Husband Ought to Know."

WHAT EMINENT PEOPLE SAY.

Chas. M. Sheldon, D. D.

"I believe the book will do great good, and I hope its message may be used for the bettering of the homes of the world."

Rev. F. B. Meyer, B. A.

"I greatly commend this series of manuals, which are written lucidly and purely, and will afford the necessary information without pandering to unholy and sensual passion. I should like to see a wide and judicious distribution of this literature among Christian circles."

Hon. S. M. Jones

MAYOR OF TOLEDO, OHIO

"I am glad to say that my study of it indicates that you have been led by a pure love for your kind to write one of the most helpful and valuable books that it has been my privilege to see in many days."

Mrs. May Wright Sewall

"It will do every young man good who reads it. To inculcate in society this sound view that knowledge upon these subjects is not only compatible with delicacy, but requisite to it, is one of the most important contemporary duties of teachers, whether in the pulpit, on the rostrum, in the sanctum, or in the class-room."

Bishop John H. Vincent, D. D., LL. D.

"Straightforward, clean, kind, clear and convincing. A copy ought to go with every marriage certificate."

Rev. Newell Dwight Hillis

"I have read your book with care and interest. It is a wholesome and helpful contribution to a most difficult subject, and its reading will help to make the American home happier and more safely guarded."

Printed in the USA
CPSIA information can be obtained
at www.ICGtesting.com
LVHW062006200823
755760LV00005B/354